HERBAL
REMEDIES
IN POTS

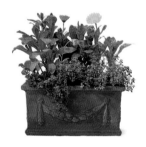

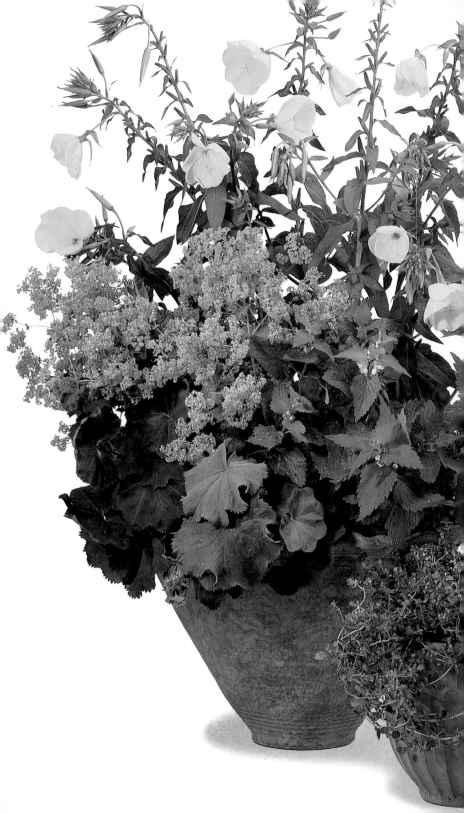

HERBAL REMEDIES
IN POTS

Effie Romain and
Sue Hawkey

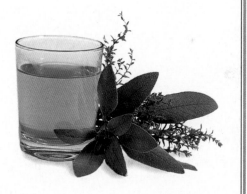

A DK PUBLISHING BOOK

Project Editor Heather Jones

Art Editor Glenda Tyrrell

US Editor Mary Sutherland

Managing Editor Maureen Rissik

Managing Art Editor Philip Gilderdale

Production Manager Maryann Rogers

Photographer Steve Gorton

Authors' dedication
For Daisy Hawkey and the Bells

First American Edition, 1996
2 4 6 8 10 9 7 5 3 1
Published in the United States by
DK Publishing, Inc., 95 Madison Avenue, New York, New York 10016

Library of Congress Cataloging-in-Publication Data
Romain, Effie.
Herbal remedies in pots/by Effie Romain and Sue Hawkey. -- 1st American ed.
p. cm
Includes index.
ISBN 0-7894-0431-1
1. Materia medica, Vegetable. 2. Plants, Potted. 3. Botany, Medical.
1. Hawkey, Sue. 11. Title.
RS164.R66 1996
615.321--dc20   95-44392
                                                                     CIP

Reproduced by Colourscan, Singapore
Printed and bound by Toppan, Singapore

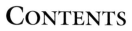

CONTENTS

INTRODUCTION 6–7

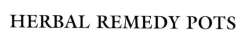

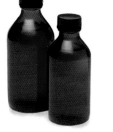

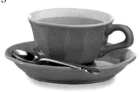

INTRODUCTION

This book is intended to help you discover the pleasure of growing some of the common medicinal herbs and to feel confident about using them in tonics or as simple remedies to treat your own, or your family's, minor health problems.

REDISCOVERING MEDICINAL HERBS

Our ancestors used herbs to treat every ailment; they had an intimate knowledge of medicinal herbs and passed this on to subsequent generations. With the advent of modern medicine, this knowledge has largely been lost. Some of the most therapeutic herbs, such as docks and nettles that bring health-promoting minerals from deep down in the soil, are thought of today only as rampant weeds and are unwelcome in the garden. Growing such plants in containers helps restrain their invasive properties, while at the same time allowing herbs that treat a particular ailment to be grouped for ease of gathering and to be grown by those with limited space.

GROWING HERBS

All the herbs in this book can be grown outdoors in temperate zones (make sure pots are frost proof to lessen cracking in winter). Some, particularly the culinary herbs, are widely available from garden centers. Many of the others are commonly found growing wild in the countryside and can also be bought as plants from herb specialists listed in local classified directories. Any plant that is difficult to obtain can usually be bought as seed.

Medicinal herbs should be in good condition and gathered at the peak of their potency. They should be planted in well-prepared soil, and watered and fed regularly with organic plant food (p.84). Keep a daily watch for pests (p.84). Never use insecticides on herbs intended for ingestion.

Annuals and perennials should be bought as small plants, or grown from seed. Some perennials benefit from being left in the pot to mature for an additional season; shrubs can thrive for years. Even if you wish to retain shrubs and perennials, clear out the pot in winter, trim tangled roots, and replant with some fresh soil mix.

MAKING HERBAL REMEDIES

Each of the 34 pots featured in this book is planted with herbs
to treat a common ailment or to provide a tonic. All the recipes
can be made safely at home, using standard kitchen equipment.
Step-by-step photographs (pp.88–92) show how to make herbal
preparations such as teas, decoctions, syrups, oils, and ointments.
Never exceed the dosages given for each remedy: if symptoms
persist, consult a medical practitioner or herbalist.

PROPAGATING AND STORING HERBS

At the end of the growing season, use the propagation
instructions and the checklist on page 93 to help you decide
whether to propagate a plant, retain, or compost it. To make the
most of your herbs, gather and dry them during the growing
season (p.86), and store for year-round use. If you find a suitable
remedy but can't grow enough of a particular herb for your
needs, supplement your supply with dried material from an
herbalist shop. Be careful of harvesting from the wild: legally,
in most countries, you can pick only aerial parts; make sure they
have not been sprayed with insecticides and are unpolluted.

KEY TO SYMBOLS USED ON PAGES 10–77

Remedy methods		Plant parts used
Tea or infusion	Gargle	Leaves
Syrup	Drops	Fruit
Decoction	Compress	Flower
Tincture	Wash	Aerial parts
Infused oil	Fresh leaves	Bulb
Ointment	Fresh roots	Seed
Cream	Seed	Root
		Bark

IMPORTANT NOTICE

The authors and publishers can accept no liability for any
harm, damage, or illness arising from the misuse of the
plants described in this book.

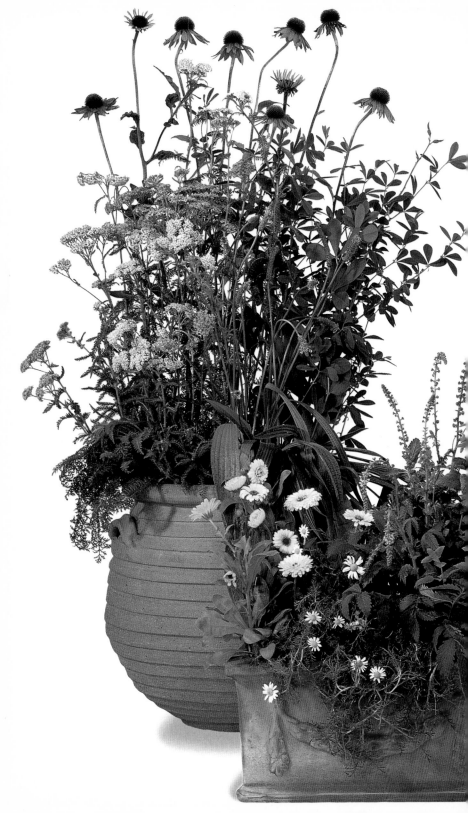

HERBAL
REMEDY POTS

*The 34 pots on pages 10–77 are planted
with herbs that treat common ailments.
There are planting and growing
instructions, information about each herb
and its therapeutic uses, and a selection
of recipes for each ailment.*

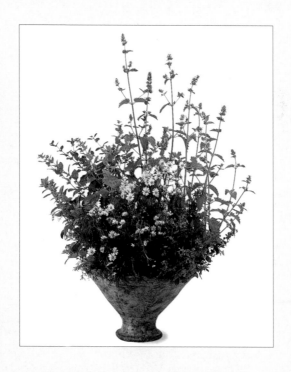

SORE THROATS, COUGHS, AND COLDS

The herbs used here contain volatile oils that clear nose, throat, and chest. Sage also has a drying effect on inflamed mucous membranes. The thymes and elecampane help eliminate sticky mucus and combine well with ground ivy and hyssop to relieve congestion.

POT INFORMATION

Herbs

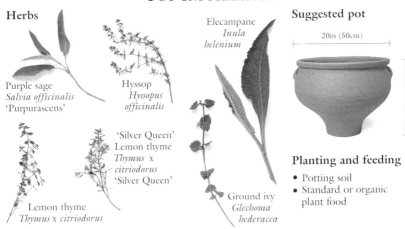

Purple sage
Salvia officinalis
'Purpurascens'

Hyssop
*Hyssopus
officinalis*

'Silver Queen'
Lemon thyme
Thymus x
citriodorus
'Silver Queen'

Lemon thyme
Thymus x *citriodorus*

Elecampane
*Inula
helenium*

Ground ivy
*Glechoma
hederacea*

Suggested pot

20in (50cm)

19in (47cm)

Planting and feeding
- Potting soil
- Standard or organic plant food

CULTIVATION

START by buying one purple sage, one hyssop, and three thymes as plants from a garden center or herb specialist. Buy two elecampane plants and two ground ivy plants from an herb expert.
POSITION in a sunny spot.
WATER daily in hot, dry weather.
FEED every two weeks in summer.
MAINTAIN the shape of purple sage, hyssop, and thymes by trimming regularly.

GATHER aerial parts of purple sage, hyssop, thymes, and ground ivy throughout the growing season. Dry for winter use. Harvest elecampane root in autumn.
PROPAGATE sage and hyssop from cuttings (p.82). Propagate thymes and elecampane by dividing in autumn (p.83). Clear out the mass of ground ivy each year, but keep a few healthy pieces of stem with roots and replant in the pot.

REMEDY RECIPES

Sage gargle CAUTION (see opp.)
Make a strong tea (p.88) with a handful of sage leaves. Add a little honey. Allow to cool. Strain, and gargle often.

Decongestant tea
Make a standard tea (p.88) with thyme, ground ivy, and hyssop. Drink at the onset of a cold or if you are congested.

Syrup for a cough
Heat 12oz (400g) sugar in 17fl oz (500ml) water until dissolved. Add two chopped elecampane roots. Heat gently. When a menthol scent is evident, add a handful of hyssop. Cook for two more minutes. Remove from the heat and let cool. Strain, bottle, and store. Take one teaspoonful three times a day.

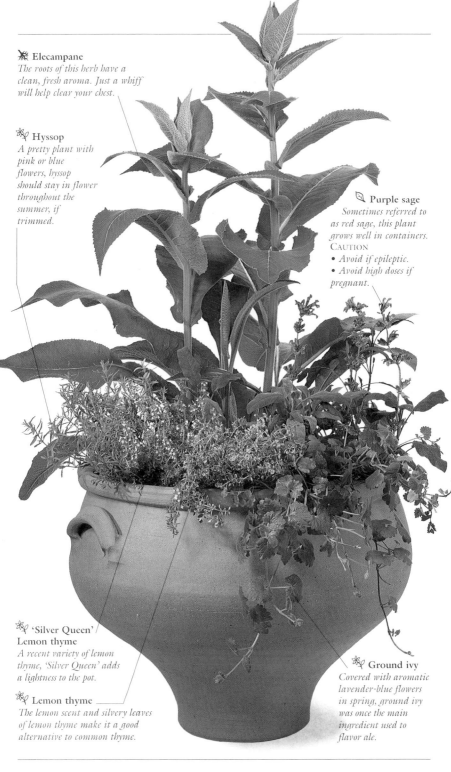

Elecampane
The roots of this herb have a clean, fresh aroma. Just a whiff will help clear your chest.

Hyssop
A pretty plant with pink or blue flowers, hyssop should stay in flower throughout the summer, if trimmed.

Purple sage
Sometimes referred to as red sage, this plant grows well in containers.
CAUTION
• *Avoid if epileptic.*
• *Avoid high doses if pregnant.*

'Silver Queen' Lemon thyme
A recent variety of lemon thyme, 'Silver Queen' adds a lightness to the pot.

Lemon thyme
The lemon scent and silvery leaves of lemon thyme make it a good alternative to common thyme.

Ground ivy
Covered with aromatic lavender-blue flowers in spring, ground ivy was once the main ingredient used to flavor ale.

FEVERS AND FLU

These herbs treat the symptoms associated with fevers and flu.
False indigo combats infection and purple coneflower mobilizes the
body's natural defenses. Plantain is astringent, reducing phlegm,
and yarrow aids fever reduction by encouraging perspiration.

POT INFORMATION

Herbs

False indigo
*Baptisia
australis*

Yarrow
*Achillea
millefolium*

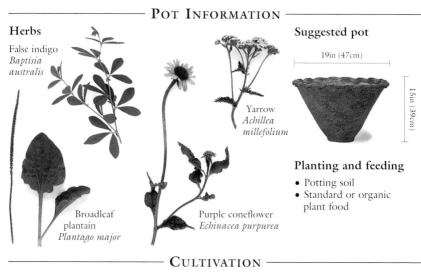

Broadleaf
plantain
Plantago major

Purple coneflower
Echinacea purpurea

Suggested pot

19in (47cm)

15in (39cm)

Planting and feeding

- Potting soil
- Standard or organic
plant food

CULTIVATION

START by buying two purple coneflower
plants from a garden center. Buy a
good-sized false indigo plant, a yarrow,
and a plantain plant from an herb specialist.
POSITION in a sunny spot.
WATER daily. Don't let the yarrow dry out.
FEED with a dilute solution every two
weeks from early summer onward.
MAINTAIN by deadheading false indigo,
coneflower, and plantain.

GATHER aerial parts of yarrow and
plantain when the plant is in flower. Dry
for winter use. Harvest and dry roots of
coneflower and indigo in autumn.
PROPAGATE plantain by detaching a
few plantlets from around the parent and
replant (p.83). Replant rooted stems of
yarrow (p.83). Divide coneflower and
indigo when they are mature enough to
provide plants for the following year (p.83).

REMEDY RECIPES

 Tea for a head cold
CAUTION (see opp.)
Most fevers and flu strike in winter, so
it is best to dry plenty of these herbs in
summer (pp.86–7). Make a standard tea
(p.88) with a teaspoon of dried plantain
and a teaspoon of dried yarrow to a cup
of boiling water. Take three or four
times a day, as long as symptoms persist.

 Decoction for flu
CAUTION (see opp.)
Make a decoction (p.89) with four
teaspoons of dried purple coneflower
root and two teaspoons of dried false
indigo root to 1 pint (600ml) water.
Strain and leave to cool. Take one
cupful, either hot or cold, four times
a day during a bout of flu.

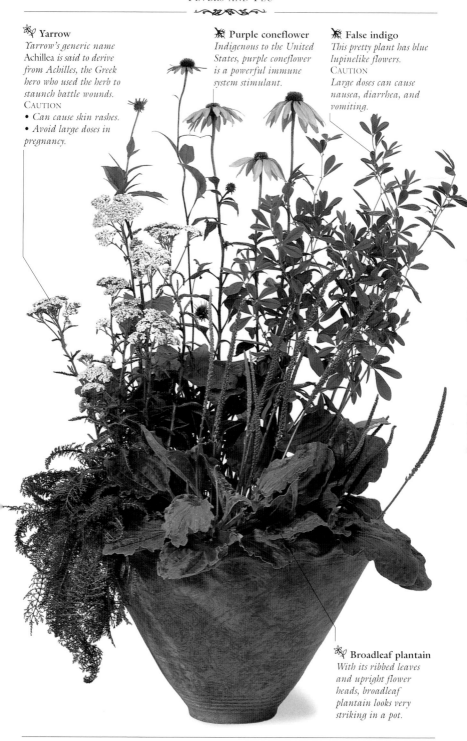

Yarrow
Yarrow's generic name
Achillea *is said to derive*
from Achilles, the Greek
hero who used the herb to
staunch battle wounds.
CAUTION
• *Can cause skin rashes.*
• *Avoid large doses in*
pregnancy.

Purple coneflower
Indigenous to the United
States, purple coneflower
is a powerful immune
system stimulant.

False indigo
This pretty plant has blue
lupinelike flowers.
CAUTION
Large doses can cause
nausea, diarrhea, and
vomiting.

Broadleaf plantain
With its ribbed leaves
and upright flower
heads, broadleaf
plantain looks very
striking in a pot.

WINTER CHILLS

*The two herbs in this pot, horseradish and nasturtium, are both rich
in vitamin C, which helps the body fight infection. They also
contain stimulating and anti-infective, mustardlike oils that make
them useful for staving off winter colds and chills.*

POT INFORMATION

Herbs

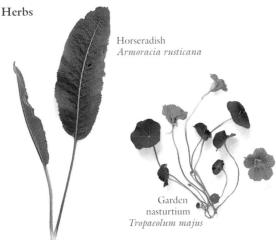

Horseradish
Armoracia rusticana

Garden
nasturtium
Tropaeolum majus

Suggested pot

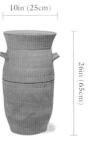

10in (25cm)

26in (65cm)

Planting and feeding
- Potting soil
- Standard or organic
  plant food

CULTIVATION

START by buying one horseradish plant
from an herb specialist in spring. Scatter a
few nasturtium seeds on the surface of the
pot in early spring, or buy four or five
plants from a garden center. Horseradish
needs a tall pot because of its deep roots.
POSITION in a sunny spot.
WATER daily in hot, dry weather.
FEED every two weeks.
MAINTAIN by trimming the horseradish
leaves if they get too straggly. Deadhead

nasturtium to encourage flowering.
Nasturtium is prone to aphid infestation:
treat any by spraying immediately with
a solution of soft soap.
GATHER aerial parts of nasturtium in the
season. Use or freeze (p.86). Harvest
horseradish root in autumn and store.
PROPAGATE horseradish by root cuttings
(p.83) in autumn. Let a few nasturtium
flowers go to seed and keep the seed for
planting the following year.

REMEDY RECIPES

Horseradish drink for a chill
To store horseradish, scrub and
peel root. Chop finely or grate. Pack
loosely into a jar. Add a little salt and
cover with white vinegar. Seal. When
needed, add one teaspoon to a cup of
hot water and drink three times a day.

Nasturtium tea for a cold
Because they are so delicate,
nasturtium flowers are better frozen than
dried. To ease colds, add a handful of
frozen flowers and leaves to 2 cups
(500ml) of boiling water. Drink one
cupful three times a day during a cold.

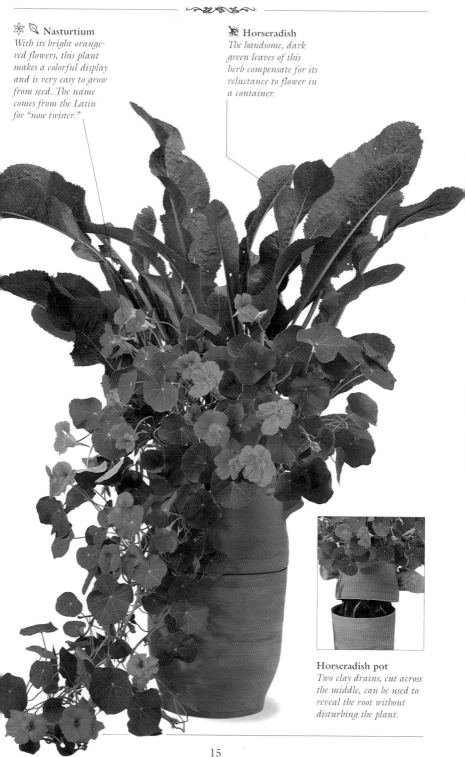

✳ ◗ Nasturtium
*With its bright orange-
red flowers, this plant
makes a colorful display
and is very easy to grow
from seed. The name
comes from the Latin
for "nose twister."*

✳ Horseradish
*The handsome, dark
green leaves of this
herb compensate for its
reluctance to flower in
a container.*

Horseradish pot
*Two clay drains, cut across
the middle, can be used to
reveal the root without
disturbing the plant.*

15

INDIGESTION

Peppermint is known throughout the world for its digestive properties. Mugwort stimulates the digestive juices, while marsh mallow soothes the intestines. Meadowsweet has aspirin-like constituents and also contains tannins, which protect the stomach lining.

POT INFORMATION

Herbs

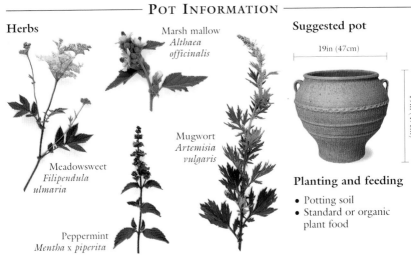

Marsh mallow
*Althaea
officinalis*

Mugwort
*Artemisia
vulgaris*

Meadowsweet
*Filipendula
ulmaria*

Peppermint
Mentha x piperita

Suggested pot

19in (47cm)

19in (47cm)

Planting and feeding

- Potting soil
- Standard or organic plant food

CULTIVATION

START by buying two peppermint plants from a garden center. Buy one each of the remaining plants from an herb specialist.
POSITION in partial shade.
WATER daily in hot, dry weather.
FEED monthly from midsummer.
MAINTAIN by trimming top leaves of mugwort to stop it from growing too tall. Use peppermint regularly in tea.

GATHER aerial parts of meadowsweet, peppermint, and mugwort as needed. Harvest marsh mallow root in autumn.
PROPAGATE mugwort and peppermint from a few healthy, rooted pieces of stem (p.83). Replant in the container. In autumn, divide root ball of meadowsweet and, if the plant is mature enough, divide marsh mallow (p.83).

REMEDY RECIPES

After-dinner tea
As a pleasant digestive after a meal, make a pot of tea (p.88) with a handful of peppermint leaves.

Indigestion tea CAUTIONS (see opp.)
Make a tea (p.88) with a sprig of meadowsweet, mugwort, and peppermint. Sip one or two cupfuls a day.

Soothing marsh mallow syrup
A syrup is a very suitable medium for this mucilaginous plant. Soak about 5in (12cm) of cleaned, chopped root in 2 cups (500ml) water overnight. Add 1 cup (250g) sugar. Heat and stir until dissolved. Simmer for 10 minutes. Strain, bottle, and store. To soothe irritation in the gut, take one teaspoonful as needed.

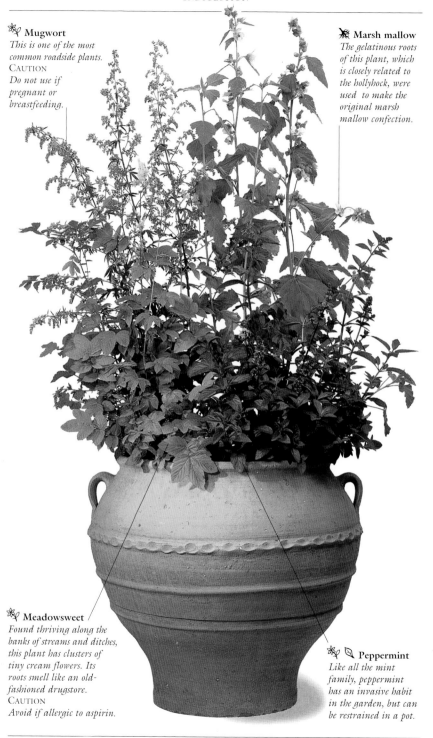

Mugwort
This is one of the most common roadside plants.
CAUTION
Do not use if pregnant or breastfeeding.

Marsh mallow
The gelatinous roots of this plant, which is closely related to the hollyhock, were used to make the original marsh mallow confection.

Meadowsweet
Found thriving along the banks of streams and ditches, this plant has clusters of tiny cream flowers. Its roots smell like an old-fashioned drugstore.
CAUTION
Avoid if allergic to aspirin.

Peppermint
Like all the mint family, peppermint has an invasive habit in the garden, but can be restrained in a pot.

CONSTIPATION

These plants will keep reluctant bowels active. Flaxseed is a bulk laxative, stretching and lubricating the gut wall. Dock roots encourage evacuation, while at the same time improving digestion. Peppermint and Roman chamomile relax the bowel.

POT INFORMATION

Herbs

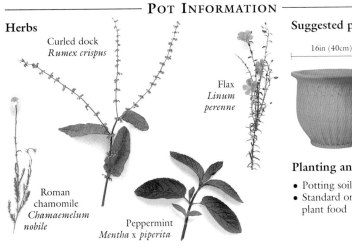

Curled dock
Rumex crispus

Flax
Linum perenne

Roman chamomile
Chamaemelum nobile

Peppermint
Mentha x *piperita*

Suggested pot

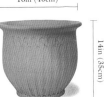

16in (40cm)

14in (35cm)

Planting and feeding

- Potting soil
- Standard or organic plant food

CULTIVATION

START dock from seed (p.80) bought from an herb specialist. Plant two in the pot. Buy five flax, two peppermint, and two Roman chamomile plants from a garden center (German chamomile can be used).
POSITION in a sunny spot.
WATER every two or three days.
FEED monthly in summer.
MAINTAIN by deadheading Roman chamomile. Use peppermint regularly in

tea. After collecting flax seed for use in remedies, cut down dead stems.
GATHER chamomile flowers and aerial parts of mint as needed. Harvest dock root in autumn. Collect flax seed as it ripens.
PROPAGATE dock and chamomile by detaching small plantlets and replanting in the pot (p.83). Propagate mint from rooted pieces of stem (p.83). Keep a few flax seed and sow for plants in spring (p.80).

REMEDY RECIPES

Flaxseed laxative
Put one or two tablespoons of seed in a cup. Add half a cup of cold water and leave seed to swell and soften. Drink before breakfast. For a milder effect, add half a tablespoon of seed to a portion of muesli. Flaxseed also contains essential fatty acids. It is safe to use this remedy over several months.

Dock root laxative
Make a decoction (p.89) with one teaspoon of dock root to one cup of water. Drink three times a day as needed.

Antispasmodic tea
Make a tea (p.88) with a few chamomile flowers and a peppermint sprig. Strain and drink three times a day.

Flax
Also known as linseed, flax is a fragile, airy plant with slender stems and flat, purple-blue flowers.

Curled dock
Because of its invasive nature, the dock is not a well-loved plant but its long roots bring minerals from deep down in the soil.

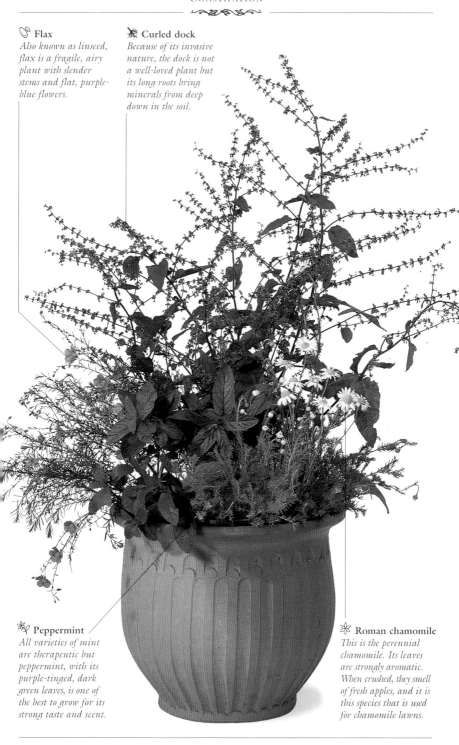

Peppermint
All varieties of mint are therapeutic but peppermint, with its purple-tinged, dark green leaves, is one of the best to grow for its strong taste and scent.

Roman chamomile
This is the perennial chamomile. Its leaves are strongly aromatic. When crushed, they smell of fresh apples, and it is this species that is used for chamomile lawns.

DIARRHEA

Containing tannins, like those present in black tea, all these herbs have a drying action, which calms and slows intestinal activity. All four are tonics, but great burnet and Solomon's seal also provide nourishment, which is helpful for digestive upsets.

POT INFORMATION

Herbs

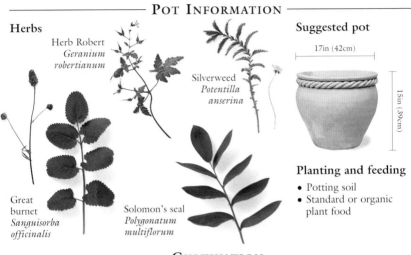

Herb Robert
Geranium robertianum

Silverweed
Potentilla anserina

Great burnet
Sanguisorba officinalis

Solomon's seal
Polygonatum multiflorum

Suggested pot

17in (42cm)

15in (39cm)

Planting and feeding

- Potting soil
- Standard or organic plant food

CULTIVATION

START by growing great burnet, silverweed, and herb Robert from seed, bought from an herb center. Plant two of each. Buy two Solomon's seal plants from a garden center.
POSITION in semishade.
WATER daily in hot, dry weather.
FEED every two weeks from midsummer.
MAINTAIN by cutting back dead stems of Solomon's seal a month after flowering. To do so any sooner will starve the rhizome.

GATHER aerial parts of silverweed, great burnet, and herb Robert as needed. In autumn, harvest root of Solomon's seal and great burnet for use (p.87).
PROPAGATE silverweed by detaching a few plantlets (p.83). Divide great burnet (p.83) and sow seed of herb Robert (p.80). New "buds" will have formed on the Solomon's seal rhizomes. For plants next year, cut out budded sections and pot.

REMEDY RECIPES

 Antidiarrheal tea
Add a sprig of herb Robert, great burnet, and silverweed to a cup of boiling water. Drink three times a day, as needed.

 Fresh root of Solomon's seal
Solomon's seal is described by herbalists as "healing and sealing." The root contains nutritious starches and can be eaten raw like a vegetable. Unearth a couple of roots, clean them, and chew during an attack of diarrhea.

 Antidiarrheal decoction
Make a standard decoction (p.89) with root of great burnet or Solomon's seal. Drink a cupful three times a day, as needed.

❉ ❊ Great burnet
The leaves of great burnet taste slightly like walnuts, and they make a pleasant addition to salads.

❉ Herb Robert
A delicate annual, herb Robert is very liberal with its seed. Its foliage turns an attractive red in autumn or in drought.

❊ Solomon's seal
In spring, creamy white pendent flowers hang from each leaf axil. Growing Solomon's seal in a container makes it easier to control insect infestations.

❉ Silverweed
This lovely plant gets its name from its silvery green foliage. Herbalists maintain that a leaf placed in a shoe will relieve aching feet.

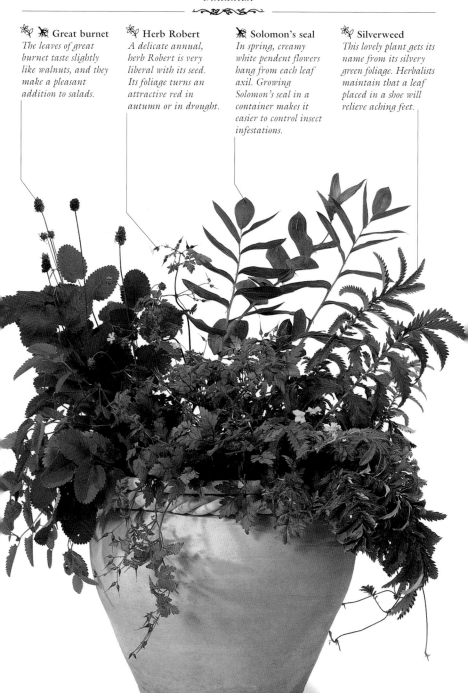

IRRITABLE BOWEL SYNDROME

Each plant treats a different aspect of this condition. Roman chamomile and lemon balm are relaxing and anti-inflammatory; the chamomile can also reduce allergic reactions. Agrimony is a digestive tonic, while pot marigold is healing and antifungal.

POT INFORMATION

Herbs

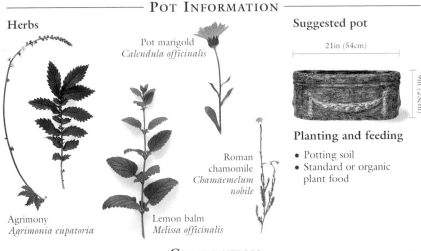

Pot marigold
Calendula officinalis

Roman
chamomile
*Chamaemelum
nobile*

Agrimony
Agrimonia eupatoria

Lemon balm
Melissa officinalis

Suggested pot

21in (54cm)

9in (23cm)

Planting and feeding

- Potting soil
- Standard or organic plant food

CULTIVATION

START by buying two plants each of Roman chamomile and lemon balm from a garden center. Buy two agrimony plants from an herb specialist. Pot marigold can be bought as plants or grown from seed. Plant two.
POSITION in a sunny spot.
WATER daily in hot, dry weather.
FEED monthly in summer.
MAINTAIN by trimming lemon balm. Deadhead pot marigold and chamomile.

GATHER chamomile and pot marigold flowers as they appear. Pick aerial parts of lemon balm and agrimony as needed.
PROPAGATE lemon balm from pieces of rooted stem (p.83). In autumn, collect marigold seed and resow for plants next spring (p.80). Propagate Roman chamomile by detaching a few plantlets; replant in the pot (p.83). Propagate agrimony by dividing the root ball (p.83) in autumn.

REMEDY RECIPES

Calming chamomile tea
Make a strong tea (p.88) with three teaspoons of fresh flowers, or two of dried, per cup of boiling water. Strain and drink three times a day, as needed.

Bowel tonic tea
Make a tea (p.88) with chamomile and pot marigold flowers, and aerial parts

of agrimony and lemon balm. Use two teaspoons mixed fresh herbs or one of dried to a cup of water. Drink regularly.

Relaxing tea
Make a tea (p.88) with a handful of lemon balm and a few chamomile flowers to 2 cups (600ml) water. Steep, strain, and drink three times a day.

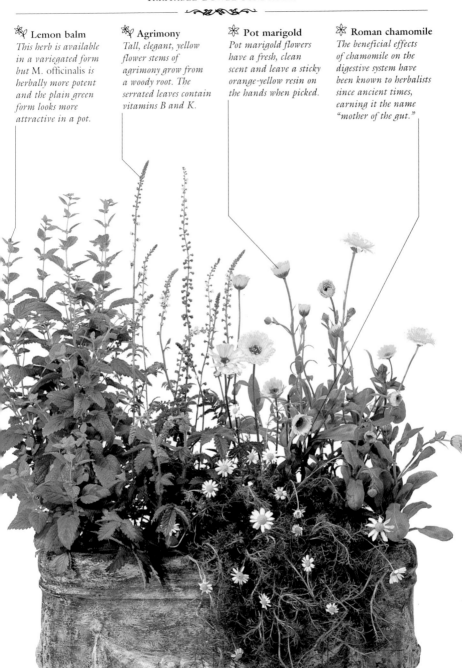

❧ Lemon balm
This herb is available in a variegated form but M. officinalis *is herbally more potent and the plain green form looks more attractive in a pot.*

❧ Agrimony
Tall, elegant, yellow flower stems of agrimony grow from a woody root. The serrated leaves contain vitamins B and K.

❋ Pot marigold
Pot marigold flowers have a fresh, clean scent and leave a sticky orange-yellow resin on the hands when picked.

❋ Roman chamomile
The beneficial effects of chamomile on the digestive system have been known to herbalists since ancient times, earning it the name "mother of the gut."

HEMORRHOIDS

Also known as piles, hemorrhoids are varicose veins in the rectum wall. Celandine and witch hazel are both astringent and will help shrink piles. Pot marigold helps reduce inflammation, and peppermint has a slight anesthetic effect and will relieve discomfort.

POT INFORMATION

Herbs

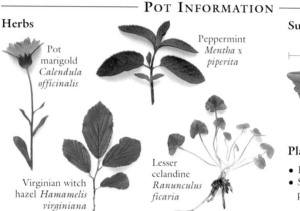

Pot marigold
Calendula officinalis

Peppermint
Mentha x piperita

Virginian witch hazel *Hamamelis virginiana*

Lesser celandine *Ranunculus ficaria*

Suggested pot

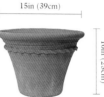

15in (39cm)

10in (25cm)

Planting and feeding

- Potting soil
- Standard or organic plant food

CULTIVATION

START by buying a witch hazel plant from a shrub or herb specialist. Grow celandine from seed bought from an herb specialist. Buy two peppermint plants from a garden center. Grow pot marigolds from seed or buy six young plants.
POSITION in a sunny spot.
WATER regularly and daily in hot, dry weather. Don't let the witch hazel dry out.
FEED weekly in summer with a diluted fertilizer– about half as strong as any recommended dilution.

MAINTAIN by deadheading pot marigold and pinching growing points of witch hazel.
GATHER aerial parts of peppermint and leaves of witch hazel as required. Collect witch hazel bark when woody enough. In summer, unearth celandine roots. Collect marigold flowers as they appear.
PROPAGATE pot marigold by collecting and sowing seed (p.80). Propagate mint from a few rooted pieces of stem (p.83). Thin celandine root ball to two roots. Leave witch hazel for three years, then divide.

REMEDY RECIPES

Pile ointment CAUTION (see opp.) Pot marigold, celandine, and witch hazel can be made into an ointment using petroleum jelly or a base cream (p.92). Chop up the witch hazel bark, the celandine root, and add to the cream. Use one tablespoon of root and bark to each cup (200g) of cream. Add four fresh or dried pot marigold flowers

and heat gently for 15 minutes. At the last moment, add a peppermint sprig. Strain into jars. Use as needed.

Tea to help piles
To treat piles internally, make a standard tea (p.88) with pot marigold flowers and witch hazel leaves. Drink a cupful three times a day, as needed.

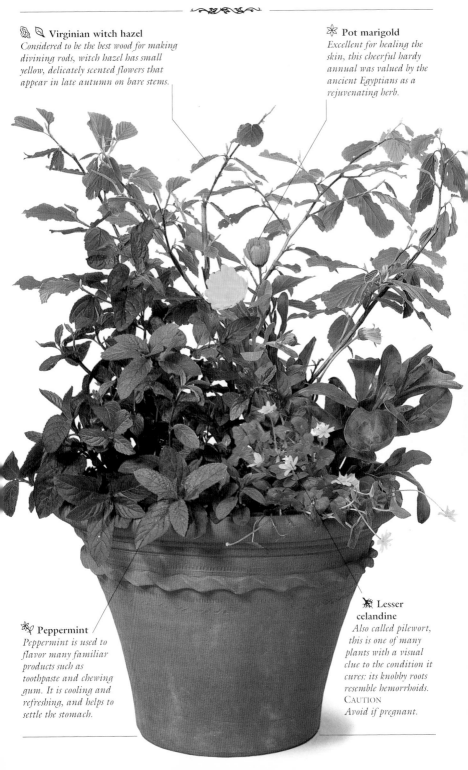

Virginian witch hazel
Considered to be the best wood for making divining rods, witch hazel has small yellow, delicately scented flowers that appear in late autumn on bare stems.

Pot marigold
Excellent for healing the skin, this cheerful hardy annual was valued by the ancient Egyptians as a rejuvenating herb.

Peppermint
Peppermint is used to flavor many familiar products such as toothpaste and chewing gum. It is cooling and refreshing, and helps to settle the stomach.

Lesser celandine
Also called pilewort, this is one of many plants with a visual clue to the condition it cures: its knobby roots resemble hemorrhoids.
CAUTION
Avoid if pregnant.

TENSION

These herbs each promote relaxation in a different way. Skullcap helps calm mental agitation, and betony relieves anxiety and tension headaches. German chamomile and lemon balm relax a nervous stomach, and lavender lifts the spirits.

POT INFORMATION

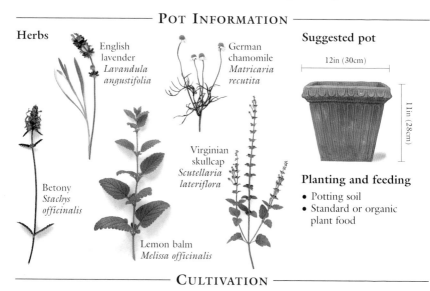

Herbs

English lavender
Lavandula angustifolia

German chamomile
Matricaria recutita

Virginian skullcap
Scutellaria lateriflora

Betony
Stachys officinalis

Lemon balm
Melissa officinalis

Suggested pot

12in (30cm)

11in (28cm)

Planting and feeding
- Potting soil
- Standard or organic plant food

CULTIVATION

START by sowing chamomile seed (p.80), bought from an herb specialist. Plant two in the container. Buy one lemon balm, two skullcap, two betony, and three lavender plants from an herb specialist.
POSITION in a sunny spot.
WATER daily during hot, dry weather.
FEED monthly during the summer.
MAINTAIN by trimming lemon balm and lavender. Deadhead chamomile.

GATHER chamomile flowers as they appear. Pick aerial parts of betony, skullcap, and lemon balm as needed. Pick lavender just before the flowers open.
PROPAGATE lavender from cuttings (p.82) and lemon balm from rooted pieces of stem (p.83). Detach plantlets of betony and divide skullcap (p.83). Collect seed of chamomile in autumn and sow for plants in spring (p.80).

REMEDY RECIPES

Tea for nervous exhaustion
To ensure a peaceful sleep, make a tea (p.88) with a handful of chamomile flowers and a small sprig of lavender per cup of boiling water. If fresh herbs are not available, use one teaspoon of dried herbs. Strain and drink three times a day over a period of several weeks.

Calming tonic tea
Make a pot of tea (p.88) with a sprig each of betony, skullcap, and lemon balm, plus one lavender flower-head. Fill the pot with boiling water. Drink a cup of this tea, hot or cold, three times a day, especially if you are feeling anxious.

Betony
With dark green leaves and spikes of lilac-pink flowers, betony combines well with the other plants in this pot.

Lemon balm
A bushy plant, with lemon-scented foliage and white or yellow flowers in summer, lemon balm is very attractive to bees.

German chamomile
This variety of chamomile is an annual. The scented, conical, yellow flowers contain the plant's medicinal properties.

Virginian skullcap
Handsome and particularly pest-resistant, skullcap has been used as a headache remedy since Roman times.

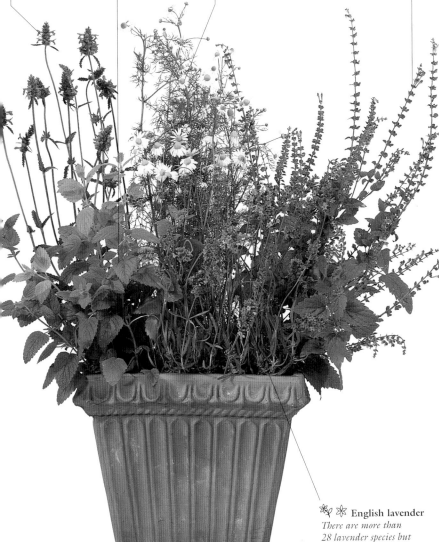

English lavender
There are more than 28 lavender species but L. angustifolia is the most potent for herbal medicinal purposes.

INSOMNIA

To find which suits you best, try these herbal sedatives. German chamomile calms the digestive system and combines well with hops, which contain sedative volatile oils. The poppy is a mild painkiller, and valerian promotes deep sleep without a hangover.

POT INFORMATION

Herbs

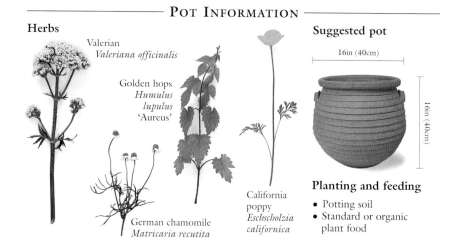

Valerian
Valeriana officinalis

Golden hops
*Humulus
lupulus*
'Aureus'

German chamomile
Matricaria recutita

California
poppy
*Eschscholzia
californica*

Suggested pot

16in (40cm)

16in (40cm)

Planting and feeding

- Potting soil
- Standard or organic plant food

CULTIVATION

START by buying four German chamomile plants, a wild "female" hop plant, and two valerian plants from an herb specialist. Because the hops will not flower until they are at least three years old, try to buy a mature plant. California poppy grows readily from seed sown in spring.
POSITION in a sunny spot.
FEED every two weeks in summer.
WATER daily in hot weather.
MAINTAIN by deadheading chamomile to encourage flowering.

GATHER chamomile flowers as they open. Pick aerial parts of poppy as needed. Pick hop flowers (strobiles) when they appear, and harvest valerian root in autumn.
PROPAGATE California poppy and German chamomile by collecting seed in autumn and sow for plants in spring. Remove valerian and hops from the pot. Separate roots carefully. Replant hops and divide valerian (p.83). When the hops are at least three years old, propagate by pulling off a side stem with roots (p.83).

REMEDY RECIPES

Sleepy tea CAUTION (see opp.)
To treat insomnia together with headache, restlessness, and digestive upsets, make a bedtime drink with a teaspoon of dried chamomile flowers and two or three hop strobiles to a cup of boiling water.

 Deep-sleep decoction
CAUTION (see opp.)
If insomnia persists, make a decoction (p.89) using a teaspoon of dried valerian root to ¾ cup (200ml) of water. Add a teaspoon of chamomile flowers. Strain. If in pain, add one teaspoon of dried poppy.

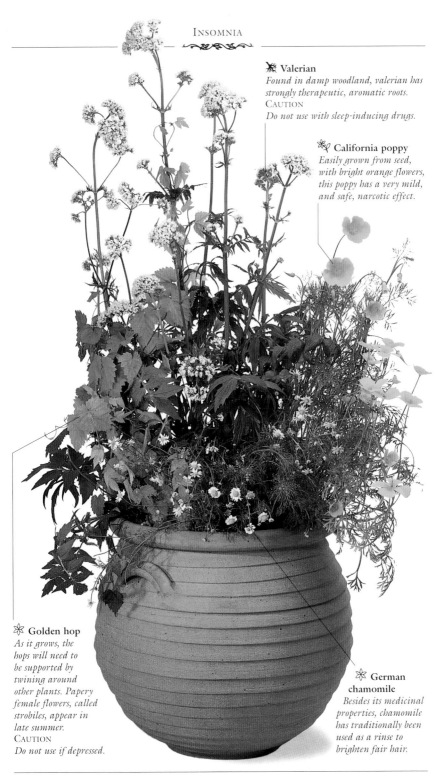

✿ Valerian
Found in damp woodland, valerian has strongly therapeutic, aromatic roots.
CAUTION
Do not use with sleep-inducing drugs.

✿ California poppy
Easily grown from seed, with bright orange flowers, this poppy has a very mild, and safe, narcotic effect.

✿ Golden hop
As it grows, the hops will need to be supported by twining around other plants. Papery female flowers, called strobiles, appear in late summer.
CAUTION
Do not use if depressed.

✿ German chamomile
Besides its medicinal properties, chamomile has traditionally been used as a rinse to brighten fair hair.

DEPRESSION

*The dull feeling of depression can be alleviated by using these herbs.
St. John's wort was a traditional remedy for melancholia, and
betony restores the nervous system and relieves tension. Lemon balm
and lavender have volatile oils that promote relaxation.*

POT INFORMATION

Herbs

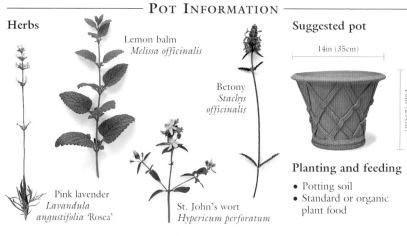

Lemon balm
Melissa officinalis

Betony
*Stachys
officinalis*

Pink lavender
*Lavandula
angustifolia* 'Rosea'

St. John's wort
Hypericum perforatum

Suggested pot

14in (35cm)

10in (25cm)

Planting and feeding

- Potting soil
- Standard or organic
  plant food

CULTIVATION

START by buying one lemon balm plant
and three lavender plants from a garden
center. We recommend *L. angustifolia*
'Rosea' because it has attractive pink
flowers. Betony and St. John's wort are only
available from an herb specialist. Buy two
St. John's wort and two betony plants.
POSITION in a sunny spot.
WATER daily in hot, dry weather.
FEED six weeks after planting and then
regularly every two weeks until autumn.

MAINTAIN by trimming all these plants.
GATHER aerial parts of St. John's wort as
the flowers appear. Gather aerial parts of
lemon balm and betony as needed. Pick
lavender flowers when they begin to open.
PROPAGATE lavender from cuttings
(p.82). Propagate lemon balm by pulling
away a few healthy, rooted pieces of stem
(p.83) and replanting in the container.
Detach one or two plantlets of betony and
replant. Divide St. John's wort (p.83).

REMEDY RECIPES

 Relaxing tea
Make a tea (p.88) with a large
sprig of lemon balm to a cup of boiling
water. Add one lavender flower. Drink
three times a day.

 Tea for a dull headache
Make a tea (p.88) with three
betony leaves or three flowers to a cup

of boiling water. To relieve the headaches,
which can often accompany depression,
take a cup in the morning, as needed.

 Cheering tincture
CAUTION (see opp.)
Make a St. John's wort tincture (p.90).
Take a teaspoonful three times a day for
three weeks and no more than two months.

❦ **St. John's wort**
*This ancient remedy
for melancholia was
supposed to scare away
evil spirits, protecting
those who planted it
at their front door.*
CAUTION
*Prolonged use can lead
to photosensitivity.*

❦ **Lemon balm**
*In ancient times, lemon
balm was considered
the best remedy for a
troubled nervous system.*

❦ **Betony**
*The Celts named this herb.
"Beu" and "ton" meant
"head" and "good." It
became a favorite
monastery herb.*

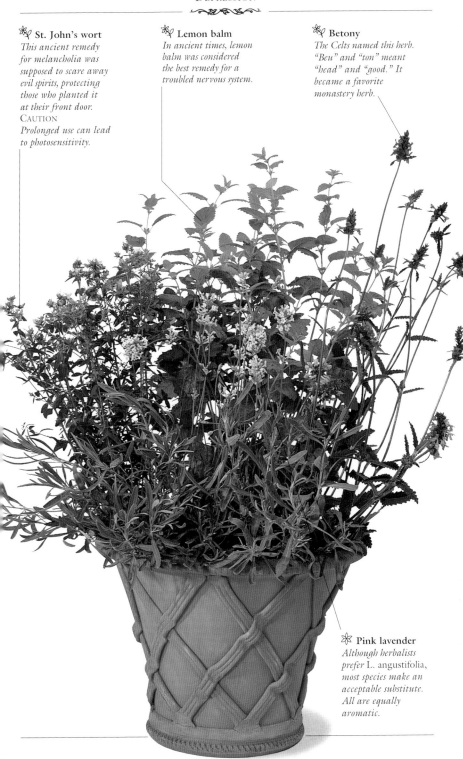

❦ **Pink lavender**
*Although herbalists
prefer L. angustifolia,
most species make an
acceptable substitute.
All are equally
aromatic.*

COLD SORES

*Caused by viral infection and linked to stress, cold sores will
respond best if treated at the first sign of irritation. Lemon balm
is antiviral, while pot marigold and garlic are both anti-infective.
Purple coneflower has beneficial effects on the immune system.*

POT INFORMATION

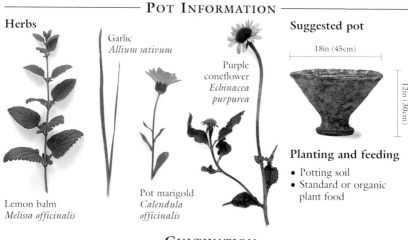

Herbs

Garlic
Allium sativum

Purple
coneflower
*Echinacea
purpurea*

Lemon balm
Melissa officinalis

Pot marigold
*Calendula
officinalis*

Suggested pot

18in (45cm)

12in (30cm)

Planting and feeding

• Potting soil
• Standard or organic
  plant food

CULTIVATION

START by planting about six garlic cloves
in autumn. These will produce plants the
following spring. Alternatively, buy four
plants in spring from a garden center. Buy
one purple coneflower and one lemon balm
from a garden center. Buy at least four pot
marigold plants from a garden center, or
grow from seed (p.80), and try to have
at least four to plant in the container.
POSITION in a sunny spot.
WATER daily in hot, dry weather.
FEED every two weeks during the summer.

MAINTAIN by trimming lemon balm.
Deadhead coneflower and pot marigold.
GATHER lemon balm leaves when needed
and pot marigold flowers as they open.
Harvest purple coneflower root in autumn.
Uproot garlic bulb in autumn or summer.
PROPAGATE lemon balm from rooted
pieces of stem (p.83). Plant garlic cloves in
autumn. Collect and sow pot marigold seed
for plants the following spring (p.80). Divide
coneflower when it is mature enough to
provide plants for the following year (p.83).

REMEDY RECIPES

Protective decoction
Cold sores sometimes appear at
times of stress. As a protective measure,
make a decoction of purple coneflower
root (p.89) by boiling three teaspoons
of root in 2 cups (500ml) of water. Add
three pot marigold flowers. Cool, strain,
and drink one cupful three times a day.

Lemon balm salve
Squeeze some juice from a lemon
balm leaf and apply directly to the skin.

Garlic salve
Cut open a garlic clove and dab
directly on to the affected area at the
first sign of irritation.

✖ Purple coneflower
*The flowers of this
plant have lovely rich
brown stamens and
purple-pink petals.
It takes several years
to grow a fairly good-
sized clump.*

✳ Pot marigold
*With their orange
or yellow flowers, pot
marigolds combine
particularly well with
purple coneflower.*

◌ Garlic
*Easily grown from a
clove, garlic has been
shown to improve
resistance to infection.*

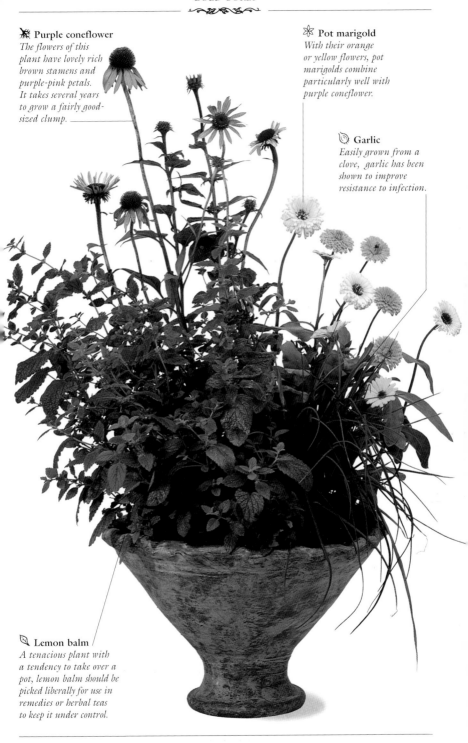

◌ Lemon balm
*A tenacious plant with
a tendency to take over a
pot, lemon balm should be
picked liberally for use in
remedies or herbal teas
to keep it under control.*

ATHLETE'S FOOT

An irritating condition, athlete's foot is caused by a fungus
that thrives in warm, damp places like those between the toes. Pot
marigold is antifungal and antiseptic, and the three varieties
of thyme have a powerful antimicrobial action.

POT INFORMATION

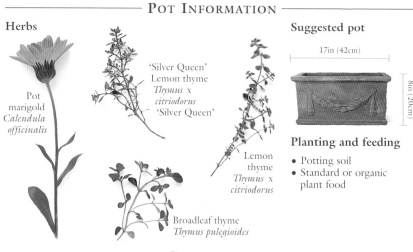

Herbs

Pot
marigold
*Calendula
officinalis*

'Silver Queen'
Lemon thyme
Thymus x
citriodorus
'Silver Queen'

Lemon
thyme
Thymus x
citriodorus

Broadleaf thyme
Thymus pulegioides

Suggested pot

17in (42cm)

8in (20cm)

Planting and feeding

• Potting soil
• Standard or organic
  plant food

CULTIVATION

START by buying the three varieties of
thyme from a garden center or specialty
herb grower. Either buy six or seven pot
marigold plants, or grow from seed in
spring and plant six or seven in the pot.
POSITION in a sunny spot. All these
plants can tolerate arid conditions.
WATER daily in very hot, dry weather.
FEED with a dilute solution two or three
times during the summer months.

MAINTAIN by using thymes regularly; trim
the plants to keep their shape. Deadhead
pot marigold to encourage flowering.
GATHER aerial parts of thyme as needed.
Pick pot marigold flowers as they open.
PROPAGATE all the thymes by removing
from the container and dividing the root
ball at the end of the season (p.83).
Collect seed of pot marigold in autumn
and sow for plants next spring (p.80).

REMEDY RECIPES

Thyme and pot marigold tea
To treat the condition internally,
make a tea (p.88) with a sprig of thyme
and one pot marigold flower to a cup of
boiling water. Drink three times a day.

Pot marigold cream
Gently heat three or four flowers
in 1oz (30g) base cream (p.92). Stir

well until the cream turns an orange
color. Strain into a jar. Let cool and
apply three times a day.

Pot marigold wash
Make a simple infusion (p.88)
from the flowers, including the outer
green cup. Let cool and bathe the
affected parts frequently with this wash.

⚘ Broadleaf thyme
This is an improved version of wild thyme. Medicinally, it is much more potent, with broader, strongly aromatic leaves.

⚘ 'Silver Queen' Lemon thyme
A relatively new variety of lemon thyme, 'Silver Queen' has random silver markings and a strong lemony scent.

✽ Pot marigold
Not to be confused with Tagetes *or French marigold, which is not therapeutic,* Calendula officinalis *is essential to any herb collection.*

⚘ Lemon thyme
With its fine, silvery leaves, lemon thyme makes an agreeable contrast with the pot marigolds.

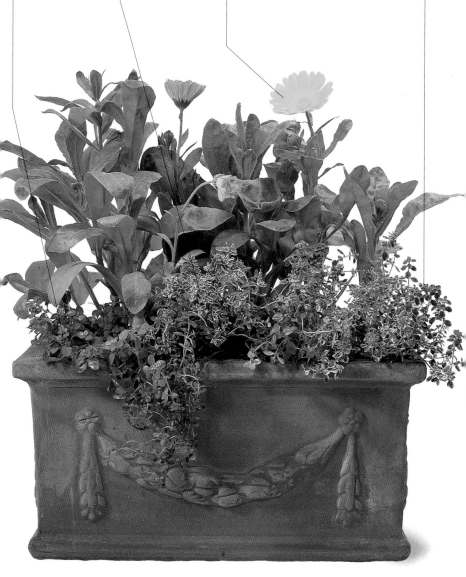

ECZEMA

All these plants are blood cleansers, helping to remove toxins from the body. Chickweed and fumitory are also cooling and treat inflamed, irritated skin. Red clover helps to nourish the skin. Blue flag aids digestion and hence the elimination of toxins.

POT INFORMATION

Herbs

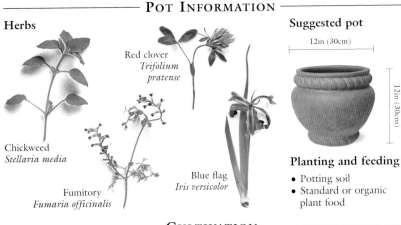

Red clover
Trifolium pratense

Chickweed
Stellaria media

Fumitory
Fumaria officinalis

Blue flag
Iris versicolor

Suggested pot

12in (30cm)

12in (30cm)

Planting and feeding

- Potting soil
- Standard or organic plant food

CULTIVATION

START by buying two or three blue flag irises from an herb specialist. Also buy three plants each of fumitory and red clover, or grow them from seed and plant three of each in the pot (p.80). When these plants are in position, sow chickweed seed by sprinkling directly on to the surface of the pot, then water. The chickweed seed should germinate in just a few days' time.
POSITION in a sunny spot.
WATER frequently in hot, dry weather.
FEED twice during the summer months.

MAINTAIN by deadheading irises.
GATHER red clover flowers when they bloom. Pick aerial parts of fumitory and chickweed when required, and dig up blue flag rhizome in autumn.
PROPAGATE blue flag by removing the plant from the container. Cut two or three budded sections from the old rhizome and replant them into the container. In spring, detach a few clover plantlets from the parent and replant (p.83). Collect and resow seed of fumitory and chickweed.

REMEDY RECIPES

Chickweed cream
Heat a large handful of aerial parts of chickweed in three tablespoons of base cream (p.92) until the cream turns green. Strain into a jar, and apply as needed. This is a good, general moisturizer. Pot marigold creams, washes, and oils, as on pages 34, 46, and 58, are also useful for treating skin affected by eczema.

Cleansing tea CAUTION (see opp.)
Make a tea (p.88) with two teaspoons of red clover flowers and a handful of aerial parts of fumitory. Drink three times a day for at least a month. To improve digestion and elimination, make a decoction (p.89) with ½ teaspoon of blue flag rhizome. Drink one cup daily for one month.

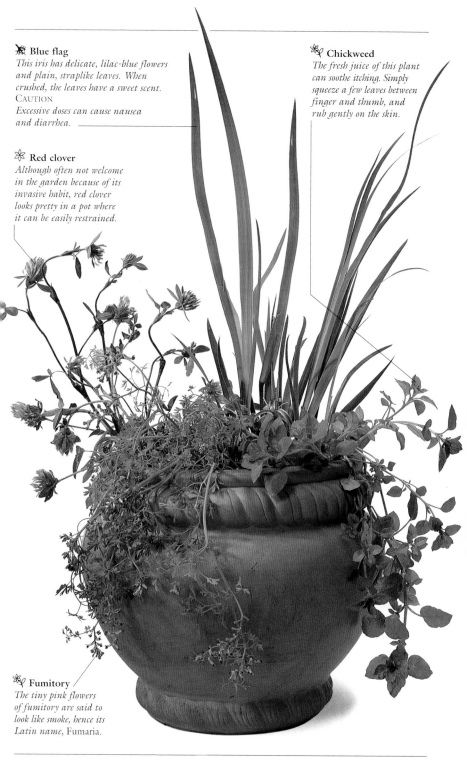

Blue flag
This iris has delicate, lilac-blue flowers and plain, straplike leaves. When crushed, the leaves have a sweet scent.
CAUTION
Excessive doses can cause nausea and diarrhea.

Red clover
Although often not welcome in the garden because of its invasive habit, red clover looks pretty in a pot where it can be easily restrained.

Chickweed
The fresh juice of this plant can soothe itching. Simply squeeze a few leaves between finger and thumb, and rub gently on the skin.

Fumitory
The tiny pink flowers of fumitory are said to look like smoke, hence its Latin name, Fumaria.

ARTHRITIS OR PAINFUL JOINTS

Herbalists believe that joints become inflamed when toxins circulate too slowly in the body. These herbs help to remedy this. Parsley and wild carrot are blood cleansers; feverfew speeds circulation; meadowsweet is anti-inflammatory, and marjoram is a general stimulant.

POT INFORMATION

Herbs

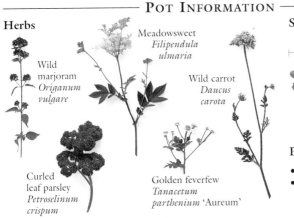

Wild marjoram
Origanum vulgare

Meadowsweet
Filipendula ulmaria

Wild carrot
Daucus carota

Curled leaf parsley
Petroselinum crispum

Golden feverfew
Tanacetum parthenium 'Aureum'

Suggested pot

22in (55cm)

13in (33cm)

Planting and feeding

- Potting soil
- Standard or organic plant food

CULTIVATION

START by buying two meadowsweet and two wild carrot plants from an herb specialist. Buy one golden feverfew plant from a garden center. Parsley and marjoram are widely available because of their culinary popularity. Plant two of each.
POSITION in partial shade.
WATER regularly and use a saucer if there is any danger of the container drying out.
FEED monthly from midsummer.

MAINTAIN by trimming all the plants in the container regularly.
GATHER aerial parts of feverfew, parsley, meadowsweet, marjoram, and wild carrot as needed.
PROPAGATE feverfew by collecting and sowing seed (p.80). Divide root ball of marjoram and meadowsweet (p.83). Collect and sow seed of biennials parsley and wild carrot in the autumn (p.80).

REMEDY RECIPES

Feverfew for improved circulation CAUTION (see opp.)
To mask the bitter taste of feverfew, put a leaf between two pieces of bread and butter. Eat daily to aid the circulation.

Diuretic tea CAUTION (see opp.)
Make a tea (p.88) with a sprig of parsley and a sprig of wild carrot to a cup of boiling water. Drink a cupful three times a day to help get rid of toxins.

Anti-inflammatory tea for pain CAUTION (see opp.)
Make a standard tea (p.88) with aerial parts of meadowsweet. Use almost boiling water. Drink three or four times a day.

Cold infused oil of marjoram
Make an infused oil (p.91) using the aerial parts of marjoram steeped in wheatgerm oil. Rub into painful joints to encourage blood supply to the area.

Golden feverfew
As it puts on growth, the golden variety of feverfew makes a bright splash of color early in the year.
CAUTION
• *Can cause mouth ulcers.*
• *Avoid if taking anticoagulants.*

Meadowsweet
The foliage and flowers of this herb have the scent of hayfields.
CAUTION
Avoid if allergic to aspirin.

Wild marjoram
With dense, pink flowers, marjoram thrives on being cut back, producing fresh, green growth until winter.

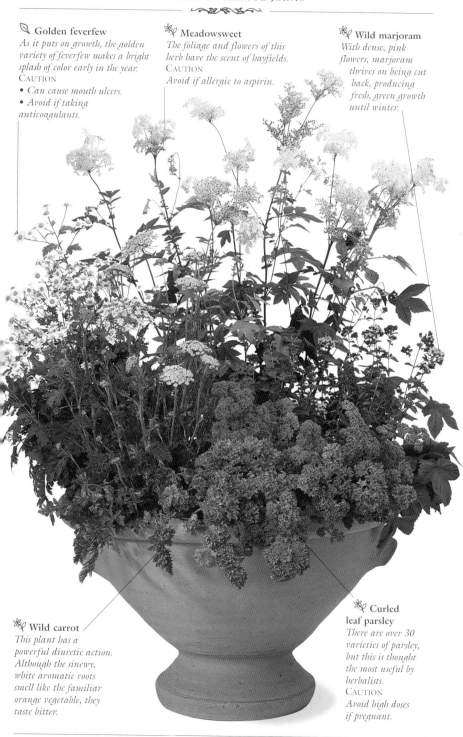

Wild carrot
This plant has a powerful diuretic action. Although the sinewy, white aromatic roots smell like the familiar orange vegetable, they taste bitter.

Curled leaf parsley
There are over 30 varieties of parsley, but this is thought the most useful by herbalists.
CAUTION
Avoid high doses if pregnant.

HEADACHES

Feverfew is known to have a beneficial effect on migraine; vervain relieves premenstrual and nauseous headaches. Skullcap and betony are nervines, with a particular affinity for the head. Rosemary is thought to improve blood supply to the head.

POT INFORMATION

Herbs

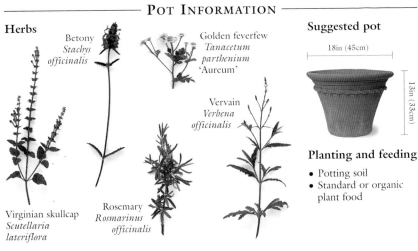

Betony
Stachys officinalis

Golden feverfew
Tanacetum parthenium 'Aureum'

Vervain
Verbena officinalis

Virginian skullcap
Scutellaria lateriflora

Rosemary
Rosmarinus officinalis

Suggested pot

18in (45cm)

13in (33cm)

Planting and feeding

- Potting soil
- Standard or organic plant food

CULTIVATION

START by growing feverfew from seed, or buy two plants from a garden center. Buy one betony, vervain, and skullcap from an herb specialist. Rosemary is widely available. You will need two plants of each.
POSITION where the pot will get some shade, especially during the heat of the day.
WATER daily in hot, dry weather; particularly watch the betony and the vervain for any signs of drying out.

FEED monthly in summer.
MAINTAIN by trimming stems and deadheading flowers. Pinch out the growing points of feverfew to encourage bushiness.
GATHER aerial parts of feverfew, rosemary, skullcap, betony, and vervain as needed.
PROPAGATE betony from plantlets (p.83). Collect feverfew seed; sow for plants next spring (p.80). Take cuttings of rosemary (p.82). Divide skullcap and vervain (p.83).

REMEDY RECIPES

Tea for tension headaches
Make a tea (p.88) using leaves from one sprig of rosemary and three leaves of betony per cup of boiling water. To retain the oils, keep the pot covered. This mixture of rosemary and betony makes a relaxing tea that will clear the head. Make and drink a cupful once or twice a day to relieve tension.

Feverfew for migraine onset
CAUTION (see opp.)
At the first sign of migraine, make a tiny sandwich as described on page 38.

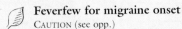

Tincture for chronic headaches
Make a tincture using equal parts of vervain and skullcap (p.90). Take one teaspoonful three times a day as needed.

Betony
In the wild, betony favors damp, cool places and tends to grow against the north- or east-facing side of trees and shrubs.

Vervain
Dense spikes of pretty, lilac-pink flowers appear on vervain in summer. In ancient times, it was considered a holy plant by Druids and Christians alike.

Feverfew
This golden variety is delightful in a pot and is just as effective herbally as the common feverfew.
CAUTION
• Can cause mouth ulcers.
• Avoid if taking
    anticoagulants.

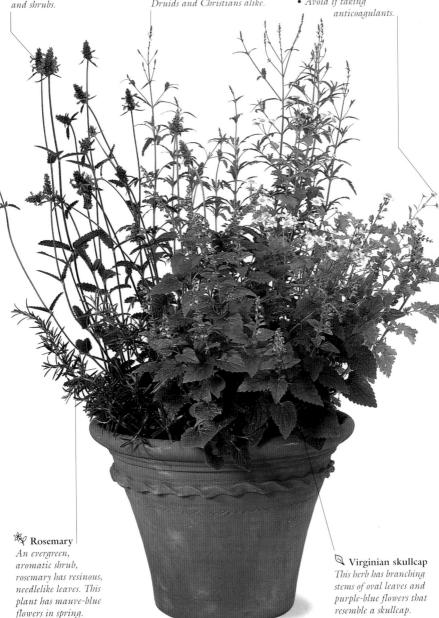

Rosemary
An evergreen, aromatic shrub, rosemary has resinous, needlelike leaves. This plant has mauve-blue flowers in spring.

Virginian skullcap
This herb has branching stems of oval leaves and purple-blue flowers that resemble a skullcap.

PMS AND IRREGULAR PERIODS

Both lady's mantle and white deadnettle are herbs traditionally used for women's problems. Taken over a few months they can help regulate the menstrual cycle. Evening primrose seed contains oils that are rich in fatty acids and reduce premenstrual syndrome.

POT INFORMATION

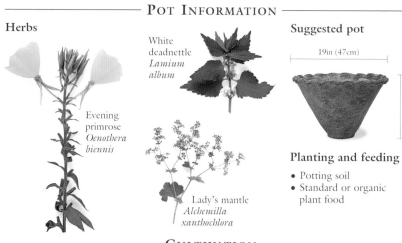

Herbs

White deadnettle
Lamium album

Evening primrose
Oenothera biennis

Lady's mantle
Alchemilla xanthochlora

Suggested pot

19in (47cm)

15in (39cm)

Planting and feeding

- Potting soil
- Standard or organic plant food

CULTIVATION

START by buying two evening primrose plants from a garden center. Buy two lady's mantle from an herb specialist. Grow white deadnettle from seed and pot four plants.
POSITION in a sunny spot.
WATER every day in hot, dry weather.
FEED every two weeks from early summer onward.
MAINTAIN by trimming deadnettle and lady's mantle and using in remedies. Keep evening primrose free of aphids (p.84).

GATHER aerial parts of lady's mantle and deadnettle as needed. Collect evening primrose seed at the season's end (p.87).
PROPAGATE deadnettle from a few rooted pieces of stem (p.83). Evening primrose can be propagated from seed, but, because it is biennial, seed sown in autumn may not flower until the second year. It may be better to buy new plants. Either divide lady's mantle (p.83) or grow from seed (p.80).

REMEDY RECIPES

Evening primrose supplement
When the evening primrose has flowered, and the seed pods have formed and desiccated, cut the flower stalks and shake the seed into a paper bag (p.87). Add the seed to a pepper mill or just sprinkle directly on to food. To help combat symptoms of PMS, take ½ to one teaspoonful every day.

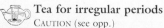

Tea for irregular periods
CAUTION (see opp.)
Make a tea (p.88) with one leaf of lady's mantle and a sprig of white deadnettle per cup of boiling water. Drink one cup twice a day for three months to balance the hormones. This can be made into a tincture (p.90) for winter use. Take one teaspoonful twice a day for three months.

Lady's mantle
One of a small number of plants that reproduces without fertilization, lady's mantle will seed itself quite freely.
CAUTION
Avoid if you might be pregnant.

Evening primrose
This is a beautiful plant, especially at night when its lemon yellow, scented flowers are at their best. The seed contains a nutritional oil.

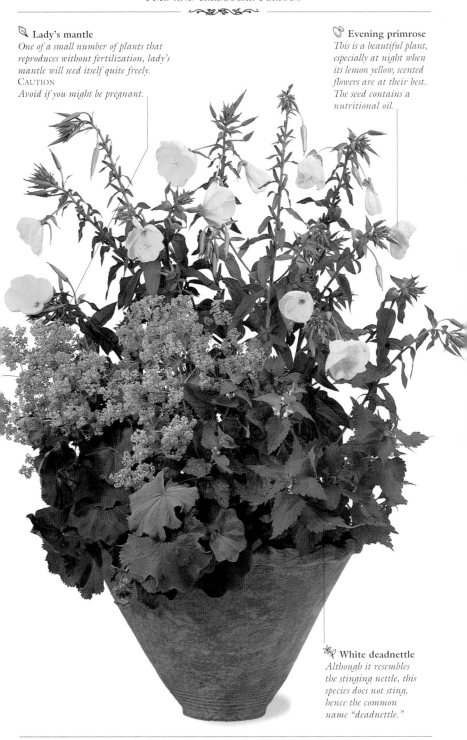

White deadnettle
Although it resembles the stinging nettle, this species does not sting, hence the common name "deadnettle."

PERIOD PAINS

As its name suggests, crampbark treats the cramps associated with menstruation. Rosemary helps by increasing the supply of blood to the uterus. Motherwort is antispasmodic and a good uterine tonic, and wild marjoram encourages menstrual flow.

POT INFORMATION

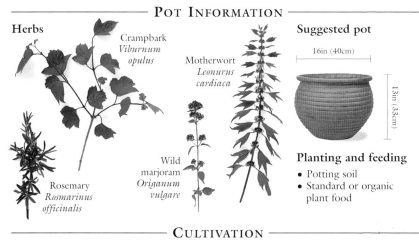

Herbs

Crampbark
*Viburnum
opulus*

Motherwort
*Leonurus
cardiaca*

Wild
marjoram
*Origanum
vulgare*

Rosemary
*Rosmarinus
officinalis*

Suggested pot

16in (40cm)

13in (33cm)

Planting and feeding

• Potting soil
• Standard or organic
  plant food

CULTIVATION

START by buying one crampbark plant from a garden center. Buy one motherwort plant and one wild marjoram plant from an herb specialist. Buy one large rosemary plant from a garden center.
POSITION where the pot will get at least half a day's sunshine every day.
WATER daily in hot, dry weather.
FEED every two weeks in summer.
MAINTAIN by pinching out the growing tips of motherwort and crampbark in spring.

GATHER aerial parts of motherwort, rosemary, and wild marjoram as required during the growing season. Use bark from twigs of crampbark after the plant has flowered in midsummer.
PROPAGATE crampbark and rosemary from cuttings (p.82). If plants are large enough, divide root balls of motherwort and marjoram in autumn and replant the healthiest pieces into the pot (p.83). This will produce plants the following year.

REMEDY RECIPES

Relaxing tea
Make a standard tea (p.88) with aerial parts of rosemary and marjoram. Drink three cups a day as needed.

Tonic syrup
CAUTION (see opp.)
Motherwort is more palatable taken in a syrup. Make a syrup as shown on page 89 using the leaves from two stems of

motherwort to ¾ cup (200ml) syrup. Take one teaspoonful morning and evening for three months.

Anticramp decoction
Make a decoction (p.89) with two teaspoons of bark of crampbark per cup of water. Bring to the boil. Simmer for 10 to 15 minutes. Drink up to five cups a day before and during a period.

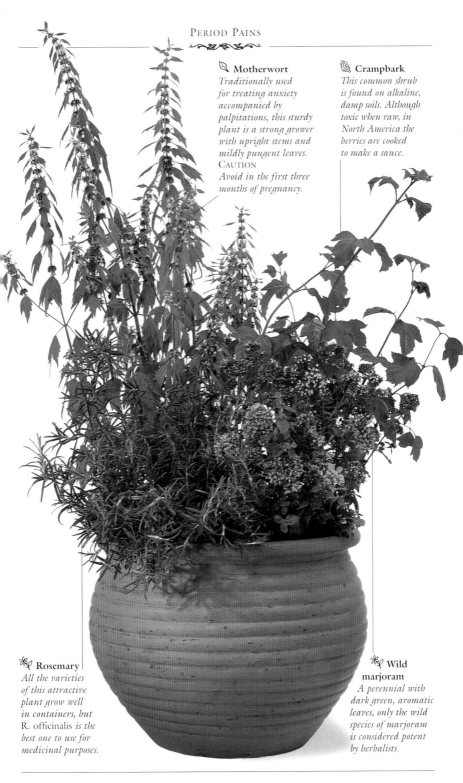

Motherwort
*Traditionally used
for treating anxiety
accompanied by
palpitations, this sturdy
plant is a strong grower
with upright stems and
mildly pungent leaves.*
CAUTION
*Avoid in the first three
months of pregnancy.*

Crampbark
*This common shrub
is found on alkaline,
damp soils. Although
toxic when raw, in
North America the
berries are cooked
to make a sauce.*

Rosemary
*All the varieties
of this attractive
plant grow well
in containers, but
R. officinalis is the
best one to use for
medicinal purposes.*

**Wild
marjoram**
*A perennial with
dark green, aromatic
leaves, only the wild
species of marjoram
is considered potent
by herbalists.*

PREGNANCY

*These herbs can ease problems in pregnancy. German chamomile
helps the digestive system cope with added demands and less space.
Black horehound reduces nausea. Raspberry strengthens the muscles
of the uterus, and pot marigold can soothe yeast infections.*

POT INFORMATION

Herbs

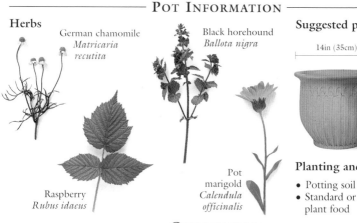

German chamomile
*Matricaria
recutita*

Black horehound
Ballota nigra

Suggested pot

14in (35cm)

12in (30cm)

Raspberry
Rubus idaeus

Pot
marigold
*Calendula
officinalis*

Planting and feeding
- Potting soil
- Standard or organic
  plant food

CULTIVATION

START by buying a wild raspberry plant
from a garden center. (If unavailable, buy
a cultivated one.) Buy two horehound
plants from an herb specialist. Grow pot
marigold from seed or buy four plants.
Grow chamomile from seed. Pot four plants.
POSITION in a bright, but not sunny spot.
WATER daily in hot, dry weather.
FEED with monthly diluted fertilizer.
MAINTAIN by deadheading pot marigold
and chamomile to encourage flowering.

GATHER pot marigold and chamomile
flowers as they appear. Pick raspberry
leaves as needed. Pick leaves of horehound
as the plant comes into bloom.
PROPAGATE raspberry by cutting off a few
suckers (new growth with roots attached)
and replanting in the pot at the end of the
season. Propagate black horehound by
dividing (p.83). Collect pot marigold and
chamomile seed in autumn and sow for
plants the following spring (p.80).

REMEDY RECIPES

 **Pot marigold wash for yeast
infections**
Make an infusion (p.88) with two hand-
fuls of flowers to 2 cups (½ liter) water.
Steep for 15 minutes. Strain and cool.
Bathe the vulva with this wash as needed.

 Raspberry leaf tea
Make a tea (p.88) with three
leaves per cup of boiling water. Drink

warm three times a day for the final six
months of pregnancy to help ease labor.
Add lemon to vary the flavor.

 Tea for morning sickness
Make a tea (p.88) with a few
chamomile flowers and two leaves of
black horehound. Stir in some honey and
let cool. Sip a cupful on waking and at
intervals throughout the morning.

Raspberry
Whether you buy a wild or cultivated one, this plant is unlikely to bear fruit in a pot. The leaves have been used for centuries by women preparing for childbirth.

German chamomile
Because it seems to have a beneficial effect on ailing plants, German chamomile is sometimes called the "plant's physician."

Pot marigold
A cold infused oil (p.91) made from this versatile plant can be rubbed into the breasts and abdomen to help prevent stretch marks.

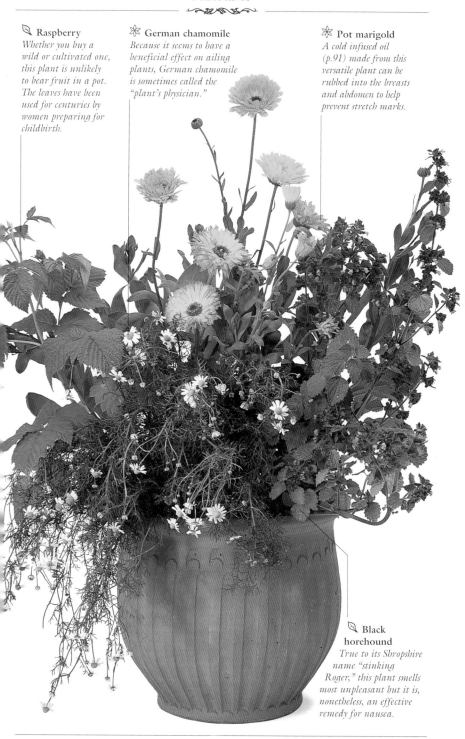

Black horehound
True to its Shropshire name "stinking Roger," this plant smells most unpleasant but it is, nonetheless, an effective remedy for nausea.

MENOPAUSE

*These herbs are women's natural allies at this stage of their lives.
Clover and sage compensate for lower estrogen levels, and lady's
mantle helps rebalance the hormones. Motherwort, a uterine and
blood tonic, reduces sweating, and St. John's wort treats depression.*

POT INFORMATION

Herbs

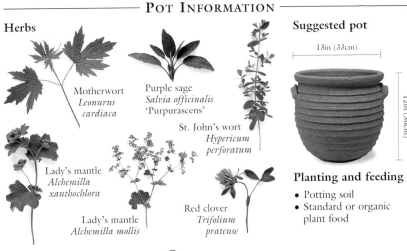

Motherwort
*Leonurus
cardiaca*

Purple sage
Salvia officinalis
'Purpurascens'

St. John's wort
*Hypericum
perforatum*

Lady's mantle
*Alchemilla
xanthochlora*

Lady's mantle
Alchemilla mollis

Red clover
*Trifolium
pratense*

Suggested pot

13in (33cm)

12in (30cm)

Planting and feeding

- Potting soil
- Standard or organic
  plant food

CULTIVATION

START by growing red clover from seed
(p.80) and pot two plants. Buy one
motherwort, one St. John's wort, and
one *Alchemilla xanthochlora* from an herb
specialist. (If you can't get *A. xanthoclora*,
you can buy *A. mollis*, but it has no herbal
value.) Buy two purple sage plants from a
garden center.
POSITION in a sunny spot.
WATER frequently in hot, dry weather.
FEED monthly from midsummer.

MAINTAIN by trimming all the plants.
GATHER red clover flowers as they appear.
Pick aerial parts of St. John's wort, motherwort, and lady's mantle when in flower.
Pick aerial parts of purple sage as needed.
PROPAGATE motherwort, St. John's
wort, and lady's mantle by dividing in
autumn (p.83). Take cuttings of purple
sage in summer (p.82). Detach a few
plantlets of clover from the parent (p.83)
and replant in the container in spring.

REMEDY RECIPES

Syrup for a hot flash
CAUTIONS (see opp.)

Chop up four leaves each of purple sage
and motherwort. Make ⅓ cup (100 ml)
of syrup (p.89). Add the chopped herbs.
Heat for 15 minutes. Let cool, then
strain. Place in a dropper bottle and take
several drops at the onset of a hot flash.

Tonic tea CAUTIONS (see opp.)
For a general tonic tea (p.88),
put two teaspoons of each herb in a
teapot and add boiling water. Allow to
steep for 10 minutes. Strain and drink
either hot or cold. A cup of this tea can
be taken up to three times a day. If
symptoms persist, see your doctor.

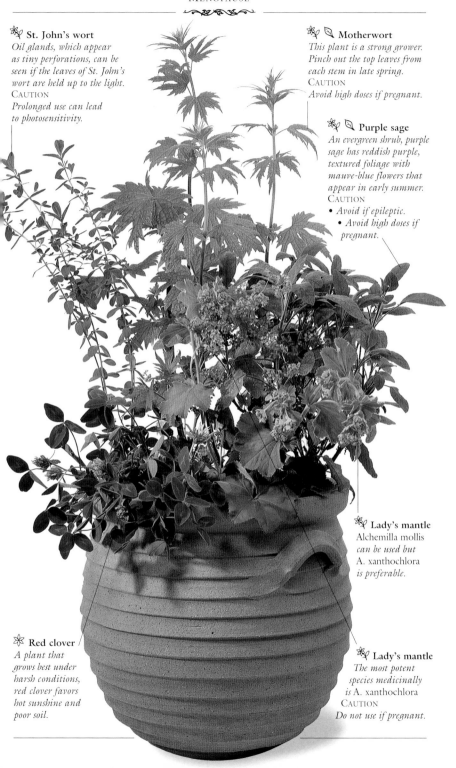

St. John's wort
Oil glands, which appear as tiny perforations, can be seen if the leaves of St. John's wort are held up to the light.
CAUTION
Prolonged use can lead to photosensitivity.

Motherwort
This plant is a strong grower. Pinch out the top leaves from each stem in late spring.
CAUTION
Avoid high doses if pregnant.

Purple sage
An evergreen shrub, purple sage has reddish purple, textured foliage with mauve-blue flowers that appear in early summer.
CAUTION
• *Avoid if epileptic.*
• *Avoid high doses if pregnant.*

Lady's mantle
Alchemilla mollis can be used but A. xanthochlora is preferable.

Red clover
A plant that grows best under harsh conditions, red clover favors hot sunshine and poor soil.

Lady's mantle
The most potent species medicinally is A. xanthochlora
CAUTION
Do not use if pregnant.

CYSTITIS

These herbs should be taken as teas to flush out the urinary system and reduce painful inflammation of the bladder. Bearberry and common juniper are antiseptics and combat infection. Heartsease and goldenrod are soothing, helping to alleviate sensitivity.

POT INFORMATION

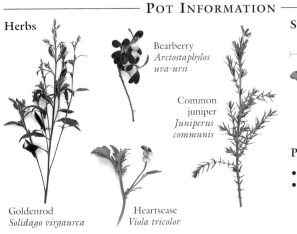

Herbs

Bearberry
Arctostaphylos uva-ursi

Common juniper
Juniperus communis

Goldenrod
Solidago virgaurea

Heartsease
Viola tricolor

Suggested pot

20in (50cm)

14in (35cm)

Planting and feeding

- Acidic potting soil
- Standard or organic plant food

CULTIVATION

START by ordering one common juniper and one bearberry from a conifer or herb specialist. Buy one plant of goldenrod from an herb specialist. Either buy four heartsease plants or grow from seed in spring (p.80).

POSITION where the container will get a few hours sunshine every day.

WATER only with rainwater if you live in an area with calcareous or limy soil. Collect rainwater in a barrel.

FEED every two weeks from midsummer.

MAINTAIN by trimming all these plants.

GATHER aerial parts of goldenrod and heartsease when in flower. Pick leaves of bearberry as needed. Collect juniper berries at the end of the summer.

PROPAGATE juniper by cuttings in spring (p.82). Take cuttings of bearberry (p.82) in summer. Divide goldenrod in autumn (p.83). Collect seed of heartsease in autumn (p.87) and sow for plants in spring.

REMEDY RECIPES

Preventive tea

Make a standard tea (p.88) with aerial parts of goldenrod, and heartsease, and leaves of bearberry. Drink one or two cupfuls per day at the first signs of cystitis.

Cystitis tea CAUTION (see opp.)

Make a tea (p.88) with one teaspoon of lightly crushed juniper

berries and one handful of mixed, fresh leaves of bearberry, heartsease, and goldenrod per pot of boiling water. If you are using dried material, use ½ teaspoon of crushed juniper berries and one teaspoon each of the other herbs. Drink a cupful about six times a day during an attack of cystitis. If symptoms persist, get professional advice.

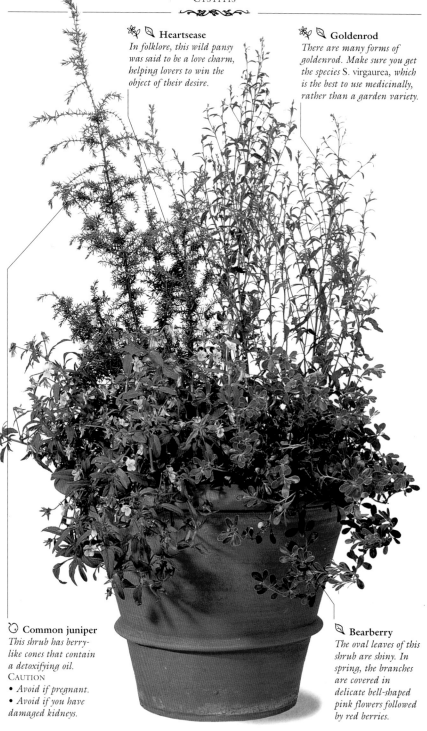

Heartsease
In folklore, this wild pansy was said to be a love charm, helping lovers to win the object of their desire.

Goldenrod
There are many forms of goldenrod. Make sure you get the species S. virgaurea, which is the best to use medicinally, rather than a garden variety.

Common juniper
This shrub has berry-like cones that contain a detoxifying oil.
CAUTION
• *Avoid if pregnant.*
• *Avoid if you have damaged kidneys.*

Bearberry
The oval leaves of this shrub are shiny. In spring, the branches are covered in delicate bell-shaped pink flowers followed by red berries.

BREAST-FEEDING

Fennel seeds and aerial parts of goat's rue are both known to aid the production of breast milk. Teas made with peppermint and fennel pass through the mother's milk and help reduce colic in the baby. Pot marigold cream eases sore nipples.

POT INFORMATION

Herbs

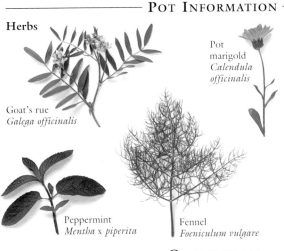

Pot marigold
Calendula officinalis

Goat's rue
Galega officinalis

Peppermint
Mentha x *piperita*

Fennel
Foeniculum vulgare

Suggested pot

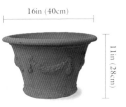

16in (40cm)

11in (28cm)

Planting and feeding

- Potting soil
- Standard or organic plant food

CULTIVATION

START by buying two peppermint, two fennel, and four pot marigold plants from a garden center. Pot marigold can also be grown from seed (p.80). Buy one goat's rue plant from an herb specialist.
POSITION the container in a sunny spot.
WATER daily during hot, dry weather.
FEED every two weeks in summer.
MAINTAIN peppermint and goat's rue by trimming and using in remedies.

GATHER aerial parts of peppermint and goat's rue as needed. Pick pot marigold as flowers open. Collect fennel seed when it forms, after the plant has flowered.
PROPAGATE goat's rue and pot marigold by collecting seed in the autumn and sow for plants next spring (p.80). Keep a few fennel seeds for sowing in spring. Propagate peppermint by detaching a few rooted pieces of stem and replanting in the pot (p.83).

REMEDY RECIPES

Tea to increase breast milk production CAUTION (see opp.)
Make a tea (p.88) using two teaspoons of lightly crushed fennel seed to one cup of boiling water. Steep for 10 minutes, then strain and drink twice a day. Alternatively, use a handful of aerial parts of goat's rue. Drink one cupful twice daily while breast-feeding.

Tea to calm mother and baby
Make a tea (p.88) with a teaspoon of fennel seed and a sprig of mint to a cup of water. Drink three times a day.

Cream for sore nipples
Make a pot marigold cream as shown on page 92. To prevent soreness, apply to nipples after breast-feeding.

Goat's rue
With lovely pink, sweetpealike flowers and finely cut blue-gray foliage, goat's rue makes a pretty addition to a pot.
CAUTION
Diabetics should seek professional guidance before using.

Pot marigold
The traditional marigold used by herbalists has single or double flowers. Double flowers give more petals to use in remedies.

Peppermint
Easy to grow in a container, peppermint has a strong taste and an invigorating, revitalizing effect, making it an ideal tea for nursing mothers.

Fennel
This familiar culinary herb has a tall habit and should be grown in a large container. The foliage, flowers, and seed all smell strongly of anise.

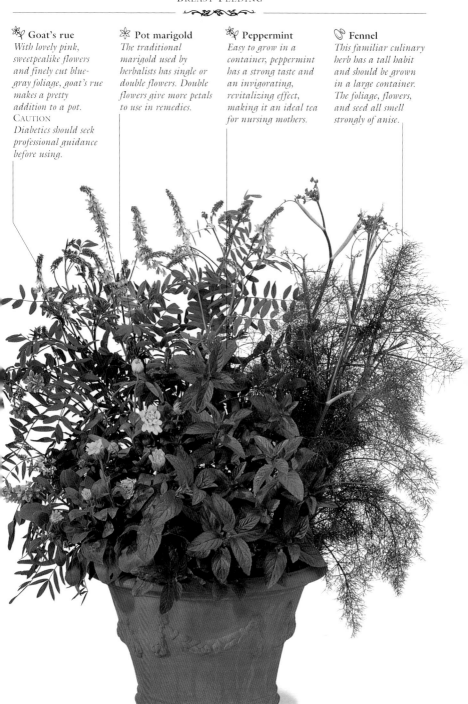

SLEEPING PROBLEMS

All gentle relaxants, the herbs in this pot are particularly suitable for babies. The remedies can be given in a bottle either alone or diluted with fruit juice. Catnip and German chamomile also help reduce fever and colic.

POT INFORMATION

Herbs

Suggested pot

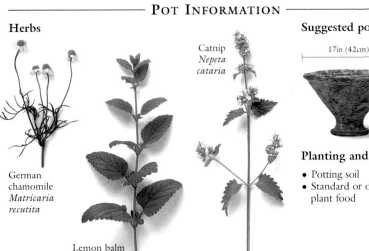

Catnip
Nepeta cataria

17in (42cm)

11in (28cm)

German
chamomile
*Matricaria
recutita*

Lemon balm
Melissa officinalis

Planting and feeding

- Potting soil
- Standard or organic
  plant food

CULTIVATION

START by growing German chamomile from seed (p.80). Plant as many as five into this container. Buy one catnip from an herb specialist. Lemon balm is widely available from garden centers; you will only need one plant.
POSITION in a sunny spot.
WATER daily during hot, dry weather.
FEED in early summer and then every three weeks throughout the growing season.
MAINTAIN by trimming all these plants. Deadhead chamomile to encourage the

plant to keep flowering. In early summer, pinch out the top growing points of each stem of catnip and lemon balm to encourage bushiness.
GATHER aerial parts of lemon balm and aerial parts of catnip as needed. Pick German chamomile flowers as they appear.
PROPAGATE lemon balm and catnip from a few rooted pieces of stem (p.83). German chamomile seed can be collected (p.87) in autumn and sown for planting in the pot the following spring (p.80).

REMEDY RECIPES

Tea to help baby sleep
Experiment with the herbs in this pot to see which one suits your baby best. Make a tea (p.88) with a small sprig of lemon balm or catnip or a teaspoon of

chamomile flowers. Strain and let cool. Dilute with 50 percent water or fruit juice and give in a bottle. Breast-feeding mothers can drink the tea to relax themselves and the baby.

✿ Lemon balm
A strong grower, with lemon-scented leaves, this herb's Latin name, "melissa," comes from the Greek for "honey-bee," indicating its attractiveness to bees.

✿ Catnip
This herb is known to attract cats and repel rats. Its spikes of aromatic pink-white flowers are also popular with bees.

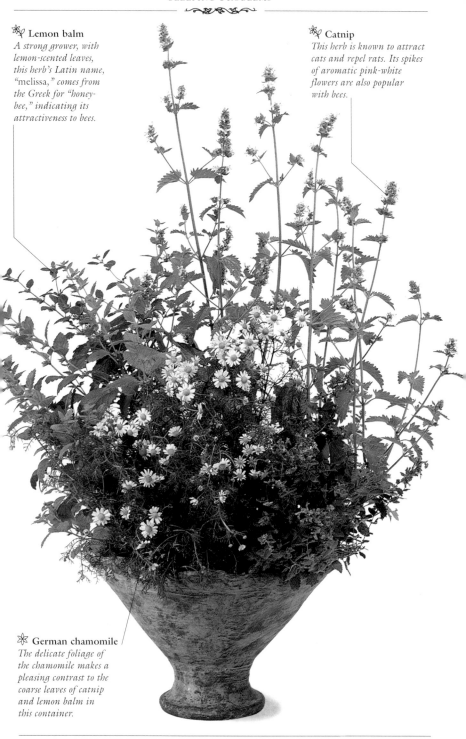

✿ German chamomile
The delicate foliage of the chamomile makes a pleasing contrast to the coarse leaves of catnip and lemon balm in this container.

STOMACH PROBLEMS

Many babies have colic, which are cramps in the stomach or intestines. German chamomile has a gentle, antispasmodic effect on the digestive system. Fennel is carminative and is used in solution to soothe babies. Agrimony is a mildly astringent tonic.

POT INFORMATION

Herbs

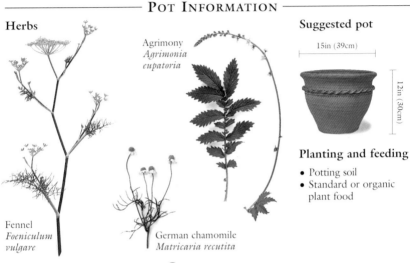

Agrimony
Agrimonia eupatoria

Fennel
Foeniculum vulgare

German chamomile
Matricaria recutita

Suggested pot

15in (39cm)

12in (30cm)

Planting and feeding

- Potting soil
- Standard or organic plant food

CULTIVATION

START by buying one fennel plant from a garden center. Grow German chamomile from seed (p.80). Plant four in the pot. Agrimony is available from an herb specialist. Buy two plants.
POSITION this container where it will receive a lot of sunshine.
WATER daily in hot, dry weather.
FEED every two weeks from early summer on, throughout the growing season.

MAINTAIN by deadheading chamomile.
GATHER aerial parts of agrimony as needed and German chamomile flowers as they appear. Collect fennel seed as it forms, after the plant has flowered.
PROPAGATE German chamomile by collecting and sowing seed (p.80). Keep some fennel seed and sow for plants next spring. Divide root ball of agrimony at the end of the season (p.83).

REMEDY RECIPES

Anticolic tea
This tea is quite safe for colicky babies and can be diluted with 50 percent water and given in a bottle. Make a tea (p.88) with a teaspoon of crushed fennel seed plus three or four chamomile flowers to a pint of water. Let it stand for ten minutes. Strain and give when cool.

Tea for an upset stomach
Make a tea (p.88) with one small fresh agrimony leaf to a cup of boiling water. Steep for 15 minutes. Strain and then let cool. Give to the baby twice a day in a bottle. If the baby's symptoms persist, seek professional advice as soon as possible.

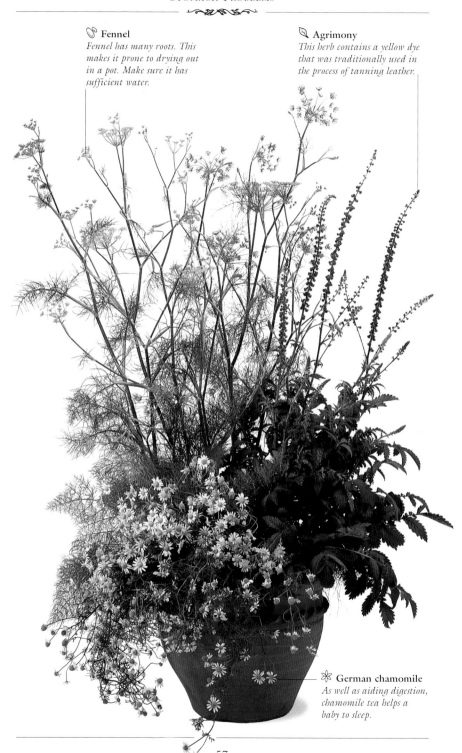

Fennel
*Fennel has many roots. This
makes it prone to drying out
in a pot. Make sure it has
sufficient water.*

Agrimony
*This herb contains a yellow dye
that was traditionally used in
the process of tanning leather.*

German chamomile
*As well as aiding digestion,
chamomile tea helps a
baby to sleep.*

DIAPER RASH

Comfrey and pot marigold are known healers of skin conditions and are suitable for a baby. Comfrey heals skin so fast that it should not be used on infected skin, since it might seal in the infection. Heartsease is soothing, and useful for treating inflamed skin.

POT INFORMATION

Herbs

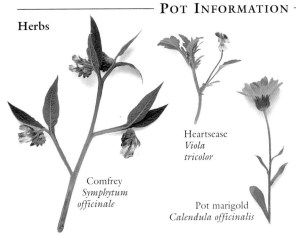

Heartsease
Viola tricolor

Comfrey
Symphytum officinale

Pot marigold
Calendula officinalis

Suggested pot

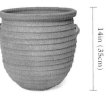

11in (28cm)

14in (35cm)

Planting and feeding

- Potting soil
- Standard or organic plant food

CULTIVATION

START by buying two comfrey plants from an herb specialist. Grow pot marigolds and heartsease from seed (p.80), or buy them as plants from a garden center. Aim to have at least four of each for planting.
POSITION the pot where the plants will receive a half day of sun.
WATER frequently in hot, dry weather. Do not allow the comfrey to dry out.
FEED monthly throughout the summer.

MAINTAIN by deadheading pot marigolds to encourage flowers. Remove large or ragged comfrey leaves and compost them.
GATHER aerial parts of comfrey as needed and of heartsease as the flowers appear. Pick pot marigold flowers as they open.
PROPAGATE comfrey by trimming the root ball to a few young roots to produce new plants. Collect seed of heartsease and pot marigold (p.87); sow for plants next spring.

REMEDY RECIPES

 Comfrey ointment
CAUTION (see opp.)
Make a hot infused oil as shown on page 91. Make an ointment by melting ½oz (15g) of beeswax into ¾ cup (200ml) of comfrey oil (p.92). Stir well. When the wax has melted, pour into jars and let cool. This ointment will protect the baby's skin. Apply on clean skin each time the diaper is changed.

Soothing pot marigold oil
Fill a jar with pot marigold flowers. Pour wheatgerm oil to cover. Seal and leave on a sunny windowsill for a month. Strain. Apply to skin as needed.

Heartsease wash
Make an infusion (p.88) with a handful of aerial parts to a cup of water. Cool to rinse the baby's bottom.

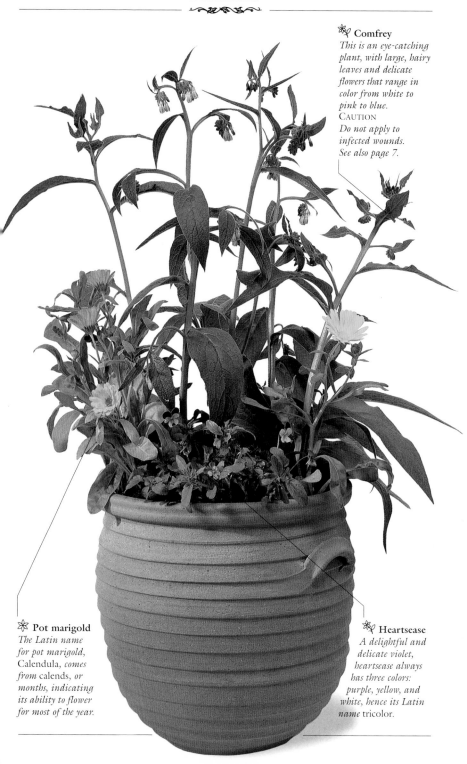

❀ Comfrey
This is an eye-catching plant, with large, hairy leaves and delicate flowers that range in color from white to pink to blue.
CAUTION
Do not apply to infected wounds. See also page 7.

❀ Pot marigold
The Latin name for pot marigold, Calendula, *comes from* calends, *or months, indicating its ability to flower for most of the year.*

❀ Heartsease
A delightful and delicate violet, heartsease always has three colors: purple, yellow, and white, hence its Latin name tricolor.

TEETHING AND EARACHE

Marsh mallow root contains a soft mucilage that soothes the irritated, inflamed gums of teething babies. German chamomile, a traditional remedy for restlessness in infants, is relaxing and carminative. Black mullein has a beneficial effect on earache.

POT INFORMATION

Herbs

German chamomile
Matricaria recutita

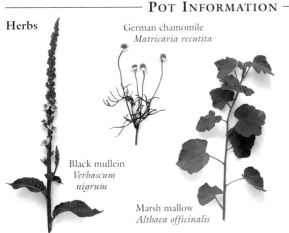

Black mullein
Verbascum nigrum

Marsh mallow
Althaea officinalis

Suggested pot

14in (35cm)

11in (28cm)

Planting and feeding

• Potting soil
• Standard or organic plant food

CULTIVATION

START by growing chamomile from seed (p.80). You will need three plants. Buy marsh mallow and black mullein plants from an herb specialist. One plant of each is enough, but several look more attractive. **POSITION** in light shade with some sun. **WATER** frequently in hot, dry weather. **FEED** monthly from early summer. **MAINTAIN** by deadheading chamomile and trimming marsh mallow after flowering.

GATHER mullein flowers as they open. Pick German chamomile flowers as they appear. Harvest marsh mallow root in autumn. **PROPAGATE** marsh mallow by dividing in autumn (p.83). Black mullein can be grown from seed (p.80) but, because it is biennial, seed sown in autumn may not flower until the second year. It may be better to buy new plants. Collect and sow chamomile seed in autumn for plants next spring.

REMEDY RECIPES

 Teething sticks
Cut and wash a 2–3in (5–7cm) piece of marsh mallow root and dry. Trim off side shoots and peel away the bark. Give to the baby to chew.

 Calming tea
Make a standard tea (p.88) with chamomile flowers. Let cool. Dilute with equal parts of water. Give in a bottle.

Teething chamomile ointment
Fill a small jar with chamomile flowers; pour on a small amount of syrup (p.89). When a tooth is coming through, strain, and rub very sparingly on the gum.

Cold infused oil for earache
Make an cold oil with mullein flowers (p.91). Strain and bottle. Put two drops in the ear three times a day.

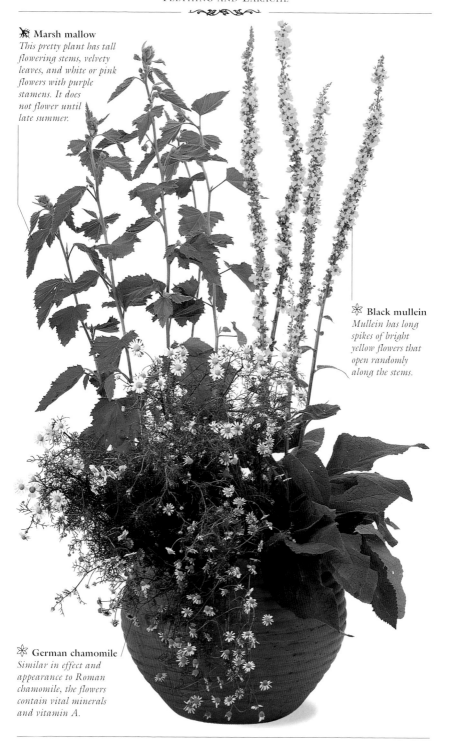

❋ Marsh mallow
This pretty plant has tall flowering stems, velvety leaves, and white or pink flowers with purple stamens. It does not flower until late summer.

❋ Black mullein
Mullein has long spikes of bright yellow flowers that open randomly along the stems.

❋ German chamomile
Similar in effect and appearance to Roman chamomile, the flowers contain vital minerals and vitamin A.

CUTS AND BRUISES

These herbs treat minor skin injuries. Yarrow stops bleeding, comfrey draws tissue together and promotes growth. Pot marigold is an all-purpose antiseptic, and arnica disperses internal bleeding and is ideal for treating bruises.

POT INFORMATION

Herbs

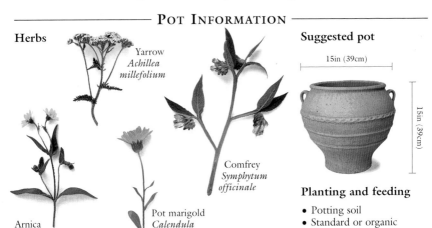

Yarrow
Achillea millefolium

Comfrey
Symphytum officinale

Arnica
Arnica montana

Pot marigold
Calendula officinalis

Suggested pot

15in (39cm)

15in (39cm)

Planting and feeding

• Potting soil
• Standard or organic plant food

CULTIVATION

START by growing all these herbs from seed (p.80). Or, buy three or four pot marigold plants from a garden center. Buy two arnica plants, one yarrow, and one comfrey plant from an herb specialist.
POSITION in partial shade.
WATER frequently during hot, dry weather. If the herbs droop, put a saucer underneath the pot, to conserve water.
FEED six weeks after planting and then monthly throughout the summer.

MAINTAIN by removing large or ragged comfrey leaves and composting them.
GATHER comfrey and yarrow leaves as needed. Pick pot marigold and arnica flowers as they appear.
PROPAGATE comfrey by removing all from the pot, leaving a few roots that will produce new plants. Propagate arnica by root cuttings (p.83). Divide yarrow (p.83). Collect and sow pot marigold seed for plants the following spring (p.80).

REMEDY RECIPES

 Ointment for clean cuts and bruises CAUTION (see p.7)
Dry six or seven comfrey leaves in a very slow oven. Prepare a hot infused oil (p.91) and use it to make an ointment (p.92).

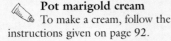 **Pot marigold cream**
To make a cream, follow the instructions given on page 92.

 Oil for bruises and sprains CAUTION (see opp. and p.7)
Make two infused oils (p.91): one of arnica flowers and one of comfrey leaves. Combine in equal parts and apply.

Yarrow juice to stop bleeding
Rub a few soft leaves together and apply the juice to the skin.

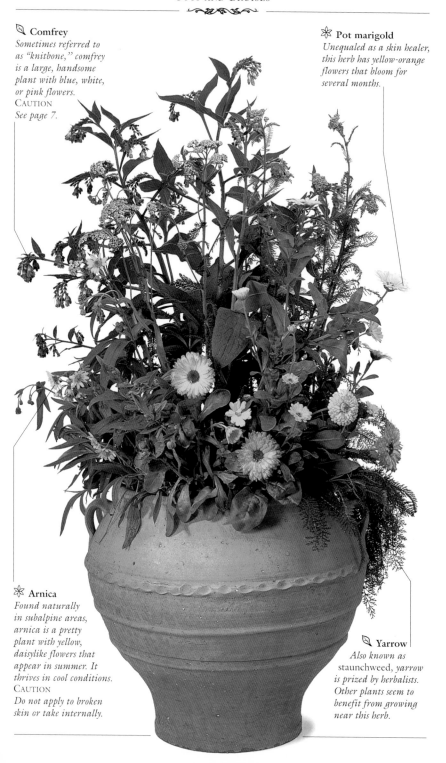

✍ Comfrey
Sometimes referred to as "knitbone," comfrey is a large, handsome plant with blue, white, or pink flowers.
CAUTION
See page 7.

✲ Pot marigold
Unequaled as a skin healer, this herb has yellow-orange flowers that bloom for several months.

✲ Arnica
Found naturally in subalpine areas, arnica is a pretty plant with yellow, daisylike flowers that appear in summer. It thrives in cool conditions.
CAUTION
Do not apply to broken skin or take internally.

✍ Yarrow
Also known as staunchweed, yarrow is prized by herbalists. Other plants seem to benefit from growing near this herb.

STINGS AND BURNS

Hen-and-chicks contains a jellylike fluid that soothes minor stings and burns, and St. John's wort heals burns. Lemon balm contains antioxidant oils to reduce inflammation. Narrow-leaved plantain and selfheal are antidotes for insect stings and bites.

POT INFORMATION

Herbs

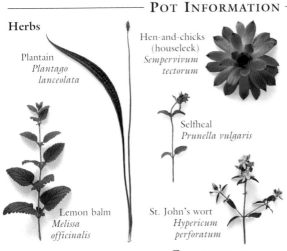

Plantain
Plantago lanceolata

Hen-and-chicks
(houseleek)
Sempervivum tectorum

Selfheal
Prunella vulgaris

Lemon balm
Melissa officinalis

St. John's wort
Hypericum perforatum

Suggested pot

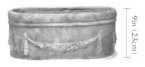

21in (54cm)

9in (23cm)

Planting and feeding

- Potting soil
- Standard or organic plant food

CULTIVATION

START by growing plantain from seed. Plant two in the container. Buy one self-heal plant and one St. John's wort plant from an herb specialist. Buy two hen-and-chicks plants and one lemon balm plant from a garden center.

POSITION the container where it will receive some sun and some shade.

WATER every two days in hot, dry weather.

FEED monthly during the summer.

MAINTAIN by trimming lemon balm during the growing season.

GATHER aerial parts of houseleek, plantain, and lemon balm when needed, and flowering tops of St. John's wort when they form. Pick aerial parts of selfheal as the plant flowers.

PROPAGATE St. John's wort by dividing (p.83). Replant rooted stems of selfheal and lemon balm, and detach plantlets of plantain and hen-and-chicks. Replant (p.83).

REMEDY RECIPES

Fresh juice for stings or burns
Pick a hen-and-chicks, lemon balm, or plantain leaf, crush and rub the juice directly on to the wound.

St. John's wort oil for burns
CAUTION (see opp.)
Make cold infused oil (p.91). Apply to area of burned skin, as needed.

Dressing for burns
Mix juice from a hen-and-chicks leaf with a teaspoon of honey. Spread on a clean piece of gauze and tape in place.

Sting and burn cream
Make a cream (p.92) with equal quantities of fresh or dried aerial parts of plantain, lemon balm, and selfheal.

Lemon balm
A generous herb, lemon balm provides leaves all through the summer. If kept in a temperature above 43°F (8°C), it will produce leaves in the winter as well.

St. John's wort
Many species of St. John's wort exist, but only H. perforatum is used by herbalists.
CAUTION
Do not go out in the sun with this oil on your skin.

Narrow-leaved plantain
This species of plantain has long, thin, ribbonlike leaves and erect flower stems that can grow quite tall.

Hen-and-chicks
Also known as houseleek, this plant needs little attention. It contains a sticky mucilage that can be rubbed into the skin.

Selfheal
The name of this pretty plant indicates its long history of first-aid use.

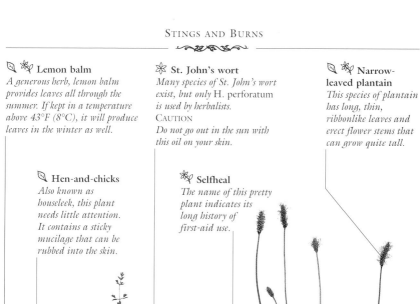

HANGOVER

Prevention is better than cure. Milk thistle tea taken before drinking alcohol in excess helps protect the liver from toxic stress. Lavender helps to settle the stomach and dispel the depression that often follows overindulgence. Mugwort is a general tonic.

POT INFORMATION

Herbs

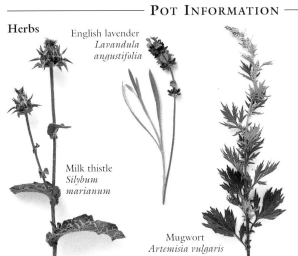

English lavender
Lavandula angustifolia

Milk thistle
Silybum marianum

Mugwort
Artemisia vulgaris

Suggested pot

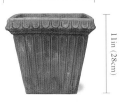

12in (30cm)

11in (28cm)

Planting and feeding

- Potting soil
- Standard or organic plant food

CULTIVATION

START by growing milk thistle from seed, or buy two plants from an herb specialist. Buy two mugwort plants from an herb specialist. Buy at least two lavender plants from a garden center.
POSITION in a sunny spot.
WATER daily during hot, dry weather.
FEED this pot weekly from early summer onward with a half-strength fertilizer.
MAINTAIN by trimming mugwort and lavender regularly. If the milk thistle leaves start to turn yellow, give the plants more water, and spray with a diluted fertilizer.
GATHER aerial parts of mugwort as needed. Collect milk thistle seed as it forms. Pick aerial parts of lavender just before the flowers open.
PROPAGATE milk thistle by keeping a few seeds and planting in the pot in spring (p.80). Take cuttings of lavender during the growing season (p.82), and divide mugwort in autumn (p.83).

REMEDY RECIPES

Preventive milk thistle tea
Make a tea (p.88) by putting one teaspoon of milk thistle seed per cup of water in a saucepan and boiling for 10 minutes. Strain and drink hot. Take a cup of this tea three times during the day before going to a party.

Liver tea CAUTION (see opp.)
Make a pot of tea (p.88) with a handful of mugwort leaves. Strain.

Tea for the morning after
Make a pot of tea (p.88) with three lavender sprigs. Strain. Drink a cup.

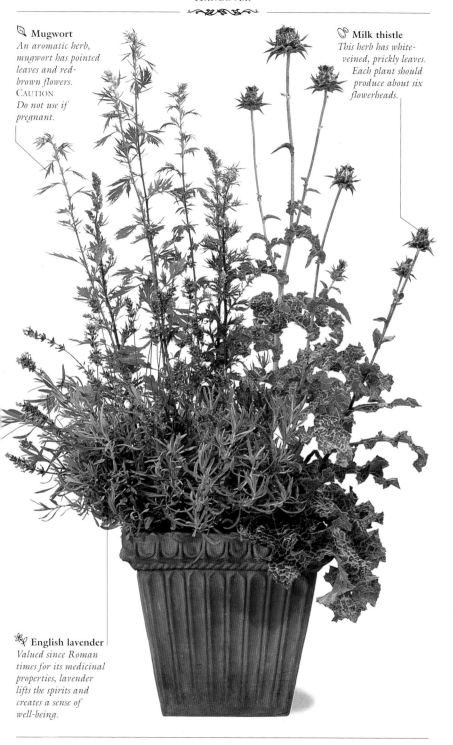

Mugwort
An aromatic herb, mugwort has pointed leaves and red-brown flowers.
CAUTION
Do not use if pregnant.

Milk thistle
This herb has white-veined, prickly leaves. Each plant should produce about six flowerheads.

English lavender
Valued since Roman times for its medicinal properties, lavender lifts the spirits and creates a sense of well-being.

MOTION SICKNESS

These herbs deal with the particular nausea of motion sickness.
Wormwood has properties to aid digestion and stimulate the liver.
Peppermint and German chamomile settle the stomach. Although
bad-smelling, black horehound is a fine remedy for nausea.

POT INFORMATION

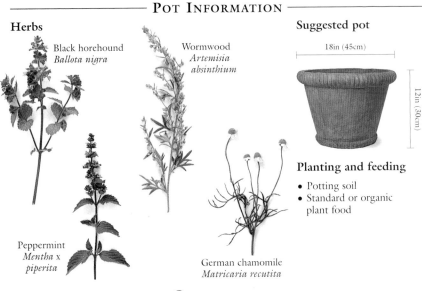

Herbs

Black horehound
Ballota nigra

Wormwood
*Artemisia
absinthium*

Peppermint
*Mentha x
piperita*

German chamomile
Matricaria recutita

Suggested pot

18in (45cm)

12in (30cm)

Planting and feeding

- Potting soil
- Standard or organic
  plant food

CULTIVATION

START by buying a wormwood and a horehound plant from an herb specialist. Buy one peppermint plant from a garden center. Grow chamomile from seed and plant three.
POSITION in sun and light shade.
WATER regularly throughout the summer.
FEED monthly from midsummer.
MAINTAIN all these herbs by trimming. Deadhead chamomile to encourage flowers.

GATHER aerial parts of wormwood, horehound, and peppermint as needed. Pick chamomile flowers as they appear.
PROPAGATE peppermint from rooted stems (p.83). The wormwood will need dividing (p.83). Horehound spreads rapidly. Divide when necessary (p.83). Collect German chamomile seeds in autumn and sow for plants next spring (p.80).

REMEDY RECIPES

Tea for motion sickness
Make a tea (p.88) with a handful of peppermint leaves and a handful of chamomile flowers. Let the tea cool. Strain and then pour into a flask. Sip at regular intervals during a long trip, or whenever you feel nauseous.

Nausea drops CAUTION (see opp.)
Steep a sprig of horehound and wormwood in 3½fl oz (105ml) of ginger liqueur. Leave for one month. Strain and bottle. Put some in a dropper bottle. Take two to four drops hourly before and during traveling.

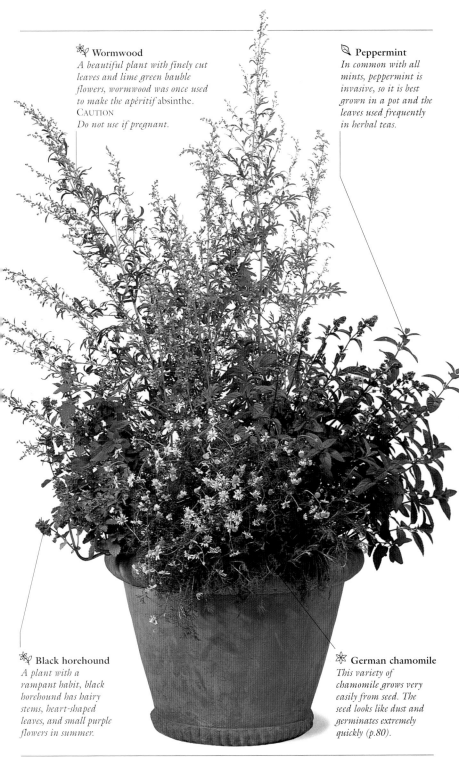

Wormwood
A beautiful plant with finely cut leaves and lime green bauble flowers, wormwood was once used to make the apéritif absinthe.
CAUTION
Do not use if pregnant.

Peppermint
In common with all mints, peppermint is invasive, so it is best grown in a pot and the leaves used frequently in herbal teas.

Black horehound
A plant with a rampant habit, black horehound has hairy stems, heart-shaped leaves, and small purple flowers in summer.

German chamomile
This variety of chamomile grows very easily from seed. The seed looks like dust and germinates extremely quickly (p.80).

NERVE TONIC

Borage is a tonic for the glands that produce adrenalin, and thus helps us to deal with stress. Rosemary and lavender are known for promoting relaxation and counteracting depression. Rosehips are rich in vitamin C, which keeps the body healthy.

POT INFORMATION

Herbs

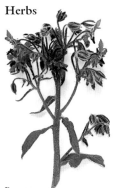

Borage
Borago officinalis

Dog rose
Rosa canina

Rosemary
Rosmarinus officinalis

English lavender
Lavandula angustifolia

Suggested pot

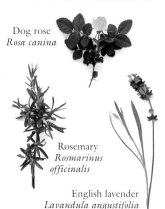

17in (42cm)

16in (40cm)

Planting and feeding
- Potting soil
- Standard or organic plant food

CULTIVATION

START by buying two rosemary plants, two lavender plants, and one borage plant from a garden center. The dog (or wild) rose can be bought from an herb specialist.
POSITION in a sunny spot.
WATER frequently in hot, dry weather.
FEED weekly with a weak solution, six weeks after planting.
MAINTAIN by trimming the lavender and rosemary. Treat any aphid infestation on the rose with soft soap.

GATHER aerial parts of borage and rosemary as needed. Pick aerial parts of lavender just before the flowers open. Harvest rosehips when they form from late summer on.
PROPAGATE rosemary and lavender by taking cuttings (p.82). Propagate the rose by removing seed from ripe hips and sowing (p.80). (Plants take up to three years to grow.) Collect and sow seed of borage for plants next spring.

REMEDY RECIPES

 Rosehip tonic tea
Make a tea (p.88) with about three or four rosehips to one cup of boiling water, then strain well. Drink daily.

 Borage tincture
CAUTION (see p.7)
Pick enough aerial parts to fill a small jar. Make a tincture by covering with

a mixture of vodka and water (p.90). This makes a gentle tonic that can be diluted in a little warm water and taken three times a day.

Lavender and rosemary tea
Make a tea (p.88) with a sprig of each herb to a cup of boiling water. Take a cupful every day as needed.

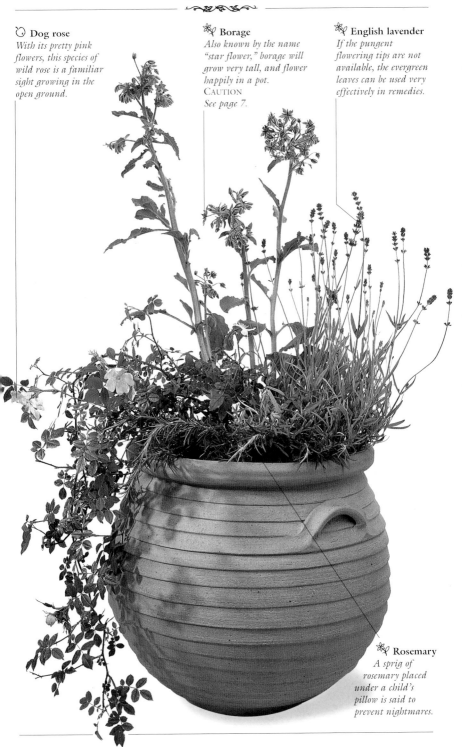

Dog rose
With its pretty pink flowers, this species of wild rose is a familiar sight growing in the open ground.

Borage
Also known by the name "star flower," borage will grow very tall, and flower happily in a pot.
CAUTION
See page 7.

English lavender
If the pungent flowering tips are not available, the evergreen leaves can be used very effectively in remedies.

Rosemary
A sprig of rosemary placed under a child's pillow is said to prevent nightmares.

CHOLESTEROL CONTROL

Garlic, wild garlic, and chives all belong to the allium, or onion, family. Known for their anti-infective properties, they also enhance the body's ability to digest fats. Southernwood, a hardy perennial, improves the liver's ability to break down fats.

POT INFORMATION

Herbs

Garlic
Allium sativum

Chives
Allium schoenoprasum

Wild garlic
(ramsons)
Allium ursinum

Southernwood
Artemisia abrotanum

Suggested pot

11in (28cm)

11in (28cm)

Planting and feeding

- Potting soil
- Standard or organic plant food

CULTIVATION

START by planting six garlic cloves in autumn, or buy four plants from a garden center in spring. Buy a wild garlic plant from an herb specialist. Buy two chives and two southernwood plants from a garden center.

POSITION in a shady spot.

WATER frequently in early spring, when the wild garlic is in flower.

FEED monthly throughout the summer.

MAINTAIN by trimming leaves of chives, wild and cultivated garlic. Pinch out topmost growth of southernwood to help maintain its shape.

GATHER aerial parts of southernwood as needed. Pick chives and wild garlic leaves when they appear. Dig up garlic bulbs for use in late summer.

PROPAGATE southernwood by cuttings in spring or early summer (p.82). The chives and wild garlic will quickly multiply in the pot. Replant new garlic cloves in autumn for plants the following summer.

REMEDY RECIPES

Southernwood tea
CAUTION (see opp.)
Southernwood has a strong, exotic flavor. To stimulate the liver and improve digestion, make a tea (p.88) using one sprig to one cup of boiling water. Drink a cup of hot tea before each main meal.

Garlic and chive syrup
Chop up two wild garlic plants, or three cloves of cultivated garlic, and two or three chives. Make 1 cup (250ml) hot syrup with the chopped herbs. Cool, strain, and bottle. Take one teaspoonful three times a day before meals.

Chives
Chives have pretty lilac flowers on long, green stems. The hollow, onion-flavored leaves aid digestion and can be used liberally in salads and as a garnish for other cold dishes.

Garlic
Familiar as a popular culinary herb, garlic can be easily grown from one clove.

Southernwood
Traditionally combined with lavender and boxwood to edge the borders of herb gardens, this aromatic herb has finely cut silvery leaves. Small, yellow flowers appear in summer.
CAUTION
Do not use if pregnant.

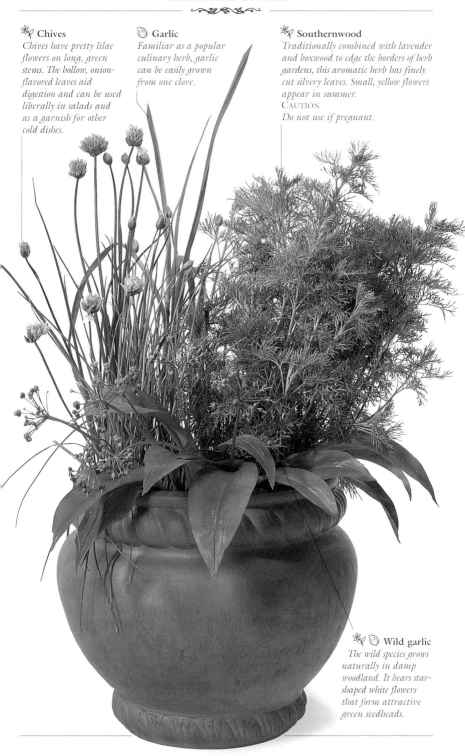

Wild garlic
The wild species grows naturally in damp woodland. It bears star-shaped white flowers that form attractive green seedheads.

VITAMINS AND MINERALS

Parsley is a blood cleanser and source of vitamin C and iron.
Alfalfa contains many vitamins and minerals including zinc, an
anti-inflammatory, which is also present in coltsfoot. Nettle and
dock are both traditional tonics because they are rich in iron.

POT INFORMATION

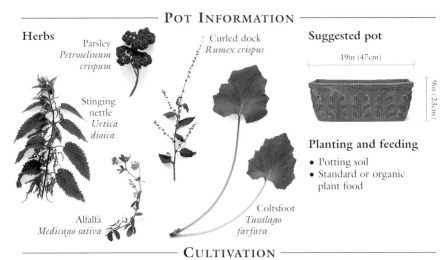

Herbs

Parsley
Petroselinum crispum

Curled dock
Rumex crispus

Stinging nettle
Urtica dioica

Alfalfa
Medicago sativa

Coltsfoot
Tussilago farfara

Suggested pot

19in (47cm)

9in (23cm)

Planting and feeding

- Potting soil
- Standard or organic plant food

CULTIVATION

START by buying alfalfa, dock, nettle, and coltsfoot seed from an herb specialist. Sow alfalfa and coltsfoot into seed trays in spring. Transfer to the pot when 4in (10cm) tall. Sow nettle and dock seed directly into the pot. Buy four parsley plants from a garden center in spring; plant in the pot.
POSITION in a shady spot.
WATER daily in summer.
FEED every two weeks in summer.

MAINTAIN by trimming nettle. Pinch out top points of alfalfa for bushy growth.
GATHER aerial parts of coltsfoot, nettle, and parsley as needed. Collect alfalfa seeds as they form. In autumn, harvest dock roots.
PROPAGATE coltsfoot, dock, and nettle by root cuttings (p.83). Propagate alfalfa by keeping a few seeds and sowing for plants next year (p.80). Collect and sow seeds of parsley, a biennial, in its second year.

REMEDY RECIPES

Nutritious alfalfa sprouts
Soak a tablespoon of seed in four tablespoons of water overnight in a jar. Pour off water. Leave in the dark to sprout for three days, rinsing twice a day. Sprouts can be eaten in salads and sandwiches.

Cleansing tea CAUTION (see opp.)
Make a pot of tea (p.88) with nettle leaves. Drink three times a day.

Tonic tea CAUTION (see opp.)
Make a tea (p.88) with a coltsfoot leaf and a large sprig of parsley per cup of water. Take a cupful three times a day.

Dock tonic syrup
Chop 12in (30cm) of root. Boil in 2 cups (500ml) water for 15 minutes. Add 1 cup (300g) of sugar. Stir to dissolve. Strain. Take a teaspoonful daily.

Alfalfa

*Although capable of
sending roots deep
down into the soil,
from where it extracts
nutrients, alfalfa will
grow happily within
the restrictions of a pot.
It has pretty, pink,
cloverlike flowers.*

Coltsfoot

*Because of its unusual
habit of producing the
dull yellow flowers before
the rosette-shaped leaves,
coltsfoot is sometimes
called "son before father."*
CAUTION
See page 7.

Stinging nettle

*Young nettle tops
can be used to make
nutritious soups.
Fortunately, they lose
their sting when boiled.*
CAUTION
*Wear gloves and use
extreme caution
around this plant.*

Curled dock

*This much-disliked
weed is rich in
nutrients. Eating
just one leaf will
give you a large
amount of iron.*

Parsley

*This popular culinary
species has densely
curled leaves.*
CAUTION
*Avoid high doses if
pregnant.*

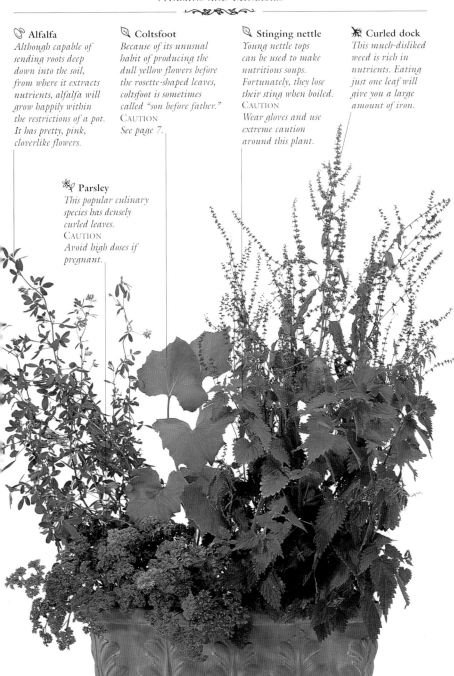

IMMUNE SYSTEM STIMULANT

These herbs stimulate the body's own defenses. Coneflower increases the activity of scavenging white blood cells, and false indigo increases the body's ability to resist infection. Pot marigold helps support the lymphatic system, and hemp agrimony is a general tonic.

POT INFORMATION

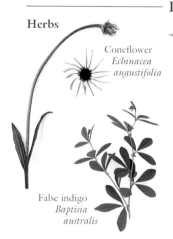

Herbs

Coneflower
Echinacea angustifolia

Pot marigold
Calendula officinalis

False indigo
Baptisia australis

Hemp agrimony
Eupatorium cannabinum

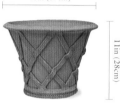

Suggested pot

15in (39cm)

11in (28cm)

Planting and feeding

- Potting soil
- Standard or organic plant food

CULTIVATION

START by buying two coneflower plants and two hemp agrimony plants from an herb specialist. Buy one false indigo plant from a garden center or herb specialist. Buy pot marigolds as plants, or grow from seed (p.80). You will need three plants.
POSITION in a sunny spot.
WATER daily in hot, dry weather. Do not let the coneflower droop.
FEED with half-strength solution every two weeks during the summer.

MAINTAIN by deadheading pot marigold and coneflower to encourage flowering.
GATHER pot marigold flowers as they open. Pick aerial parts of hemp agrimony before the flowers open. Harvest roots of false indigo and coneflower in autumn.
PROPAGATE agrimony from rooted pieces of stem (p.83). Collect pot marigold seed and sow for plants next spring (p.80). When coneflower and indigo are mature enough, propagate by division (p.83).

REMEDY RECIPES

Decoction for infections
Make a decoction (p.89) with two teaspoons of coneflower root and one of false indigo root. Simmer for ten minutes. Strain. Drink a cupful three times a day.

Pot marigold tonic tincture
Fill a jam jar three-quarters full with pot marigold flowerheads and pour enough vodka over to cover. Let stand for one month. Strain and bottle. Take one teaspoonful three times a day.

Tonic tea
Make a tea (p.88) with aerial parts of hemp agrimony. Drink a cupful three times a day, whenever you feel that you might be vulnerable to infection.

Coneflower
Similar in appearance and effect to purple coneflower (p.12), this species is probably more potent.

Hemp agrimony
A common roadside plant in temperate zones, hemp agrimony has tall stems that bear pink flower clusters.

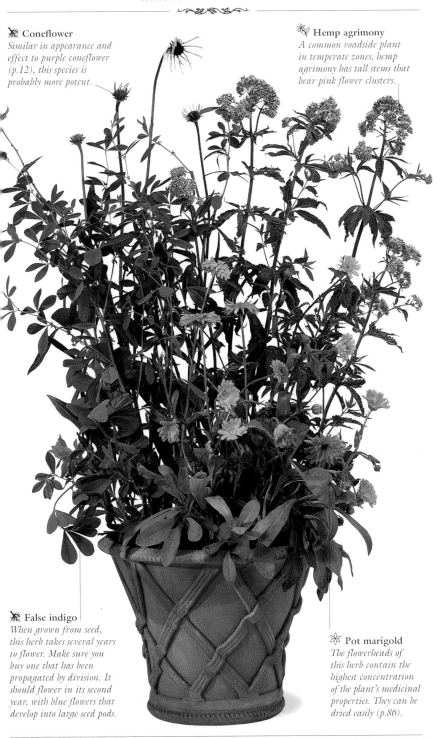

False indigo
When grown from seed, this herb takes several years to flower. Make sure you buy one that has been propagated by division. It should flower in its second year, with blue flowers that develop into large seed pods.

Pot marigold
The flowerheads of this herb contain the highest concentration of the plant's medicinal properties. They can be dried easily (p.86).

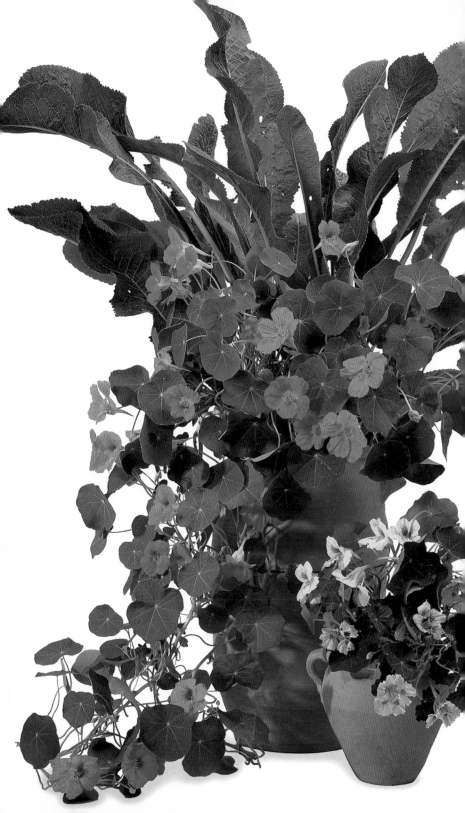

GROWING HERBS AND MAKING REMEDIES

The main methods of growing and propagating herbs – by seed, cuttings, and dividing – are shown in step-by-step illustrations on pages 80–83. Guidelines on how to plant a pot are given on pages 84–85. Pages 88–92 show how simple herbal remedies can be made with standard kitchen equipment.

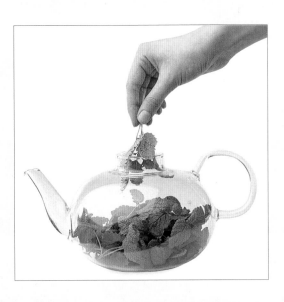

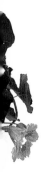

PROPAGATION

Propagating is a most satisfying part of tending plants. Before the end of the growing season, collect seedheads and take cuttings. At the end of the autumn, empty the pot: take root cuttings, divide root balls, replant perennials and shrubs.

SOWING SEED

This method is used for annuals, such as German chamomile (shown here). Whether you buy seed or collect it from your own plants, the method is the same. If seed trays can be protected from cold, sow seed in autumn for planting out in spring, otherwise sow as early as possible in spring.

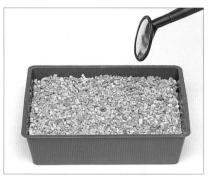

1 Fill a seed tray with a soil mix or vermiculite. Firm the surface lightly and evenly and water thoroughly.

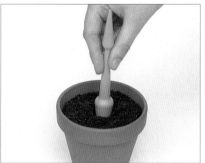

2 Sow seed on the surface. If the seed is very fine, use a folded piece of card and tap gently to scatter the seed evenly.

Remember to label the seed tray once sown.

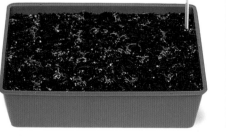

3 Cover the surface with a fine layer of soil mix or vermiculite. Position in a light, draft-free spot out of direct sun. Check the tray every day and keep the medium moist by watering with tepid water from a fine-holed watering can.

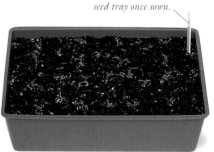

4 After three to four weeks, when the seedlings are just big enough to handle, fill as many small pots as you need plants with potting soil. Firm the surface about ½in (3cm) below the rim of each pot. Make a hole in the soil mix in each pot.

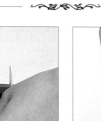

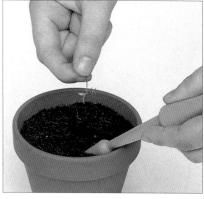

5 Gently tease out the strongest of the seedlings from the seed tray, using a widger or teaspoon. Always handle the seedlings by their two open leaves.

6 Carefully insert a seedling in each of the prepared pots. Carefully ease in the roots, then gently firm the soil mix around the seedling. Label each pot.

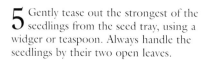

Strong top-growth indicates chamomile is ready for planting in the container.

7 Place the potted seedlings on a drip tray and water with a fine-holed watering can. Place in a light spot, away from drafts. Check seedlings daily and keep the growing medium moist.

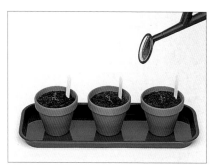

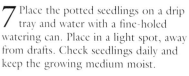

8 When the seedlings have developed more leaves, and the roots begin to fill the pot, they should be planted out into bigger pots. If they have been in a warm place indoors, expose them gradually to outdoor temperatures, once the danger of frost has passed.

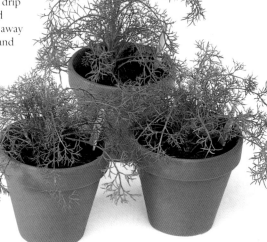

TAKING CUTTINGS

Propagation by cuttings is the best method for shrubby plants such as lavender, rosemary, thyme, and southernwood. Cuttings should be taken from healthy, nonflowering shoots during the growing season. Let root and grow on, and plant in a container the following spring.

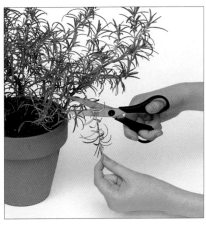

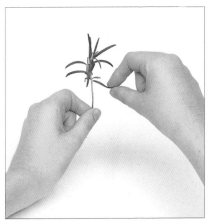

1 Select four or five healthy stems. Cut off pieces of stem about the length of a finger with scissors or small pruners.

2 Pull off all but the topmost foliage to leave a bare stem. Make a clean cut across the stem just below a leaf joint.

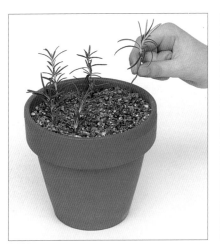

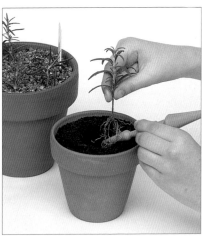

3 Poke in the cuttings around the edge of a 5½in (14cm) pot of a half and half sand-and-vermiculite mixture. Water. Leave in a light, draft-free place. After 2–4 weeks, gently pull at a cutting. If you feel resistance, roots have formed; if not, leave for a week.

4 Pot each rooted cutting into a 3½in (9cm) pot of growing medium; label. Overwinter in a sheltered position. In spring, the cuttings should be ready for planting in the container. If the plants were in a warm place, harden off before planting.

ROOT CUTTINGS

The stock of some perennials such as horseradish, comfrey, and elecampane can be increased by taking root cuttings. Do this in the autumn to obtain plants for the following spring. Remove the parent plant from the container and trim off some healthy roots with scissors.

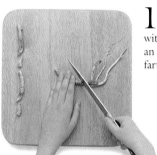

1 Cut four or five finger-length sections of root with a sharp knife, making an angled cut at the end farthest from the plant.

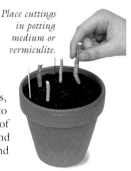

Place cuttings in potting medium or vermiculite.

2 Poke in the cuttings, angled end first, into holes around the edge of the pot. Water, label, and put out of direct sun and drafts. Keep moist.

PLANTLETS

Betony, plantain, Roman chamomile, and lady's mantle all form young plants around the base of the parent plant. When you empty the pot at the end of the growing season, gently detach these plantlets from the parent root ball. Pot, water, and keep in a sheltered position until next spring.

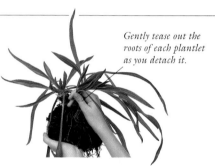

Gently tease out the roots of each plantlet as you detach it.

ROOTED STEMS

Some plants like mint and ground ivy produce new roots and shoots from stems during the growing season. Cut these root-bearing stems from the parent. Pot rooted stems of pot-bound plants like the one below, and compost the parent plant.

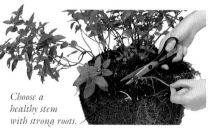

Choose a healthy stem with strong roots.

DIVIDING A ROOT BALL

Some perennials, like coneflowers, take several seasons to mature. When they do become too large, lift and divide them. Shake the soil from the roots and cut through them to obtain two or more sections. Replant to grow into good-sized plants for next year.

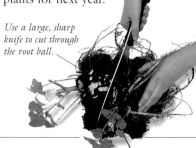

Use a large, sharp knife to cut through the root ball.

MAKING UP A POT

*Besides looking attractive, containers are a convenient
way of growing some invasive plants such as peppermint,
coltsfoot, and nettles, which would otherwise spread quickly
through open soil and soon become a nuisance in the garden.*

Growing medium
Container plants need a well-balanced
growing medium, based on soil or a
peat substitute, with lots of organic
matter. You can buy ready-made
potting soil or make your own. A
dark, crumbly soil, not sticky clay, is
best. The quantities below will fill a
16in (40cm) by 12in (30cm) deep pot.

- 1 bucket (18 liters) sieved garden soil
- ¼ bucket horticultural grit or coarse sand
- ¾ bucket leaf mold or garden compost
- 1 tablespoon bonemeal
- 2 teaspoons seaweed meal
- 2 teaspoons calcified seaweed

Sift the soil and spread in a circle,
32in (80cm) in diameter, near the
pot. Spread the other ingredients
evenly over the soil. Scrape into a
heap. Fill the pot with the mixture.

Watering
Regularly soak the soil with a watering
can or hose during the growing season.

Feeding
The nutrients in any soil mix will
need replenishing six weeks after
planting, and regularly during the
growing season. Any standard plant
food can be used, but organic feeds
such as seaweed extract or worm
castings are preferable for herbs.

Maintaining
Trim off excessive growth during the
growing season. Deadhead flowers
that have not been picked for use in
remedies or for drying, so that more
flowers form. Watch out for aphids,
and spray with a solution of soft soap,
available from garden centers.

DESIGNING A POT
Remember to decide where you want to position
your container, whether in full or partial sun or
shade, before filling it with soil mix and plants.
It will be quite heavy
to move afterward.

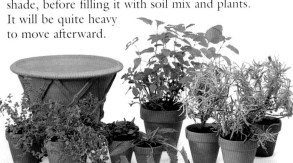

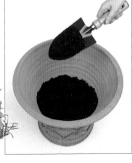

1 Assemble the plants. Put
a few small stones over
the drainage hole in the pot
and half-fill with soil mix.

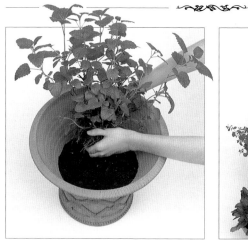

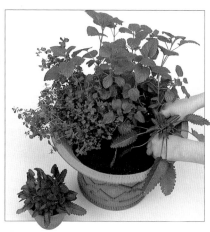

2 Choose a large perennial plant for the center of the planting so it can have as much root space as possible. Tap it out of its pot, tease out the roots a little, and place it on the growing surface.

3 Add enough soil mix to fill three-quarters of the pot. Use a trowel to make hollows in the mix around the central plant, and insert the other plants, with the larger-growing plants at the back.

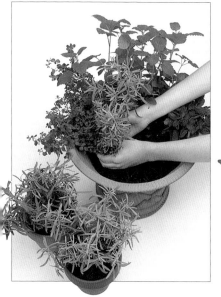

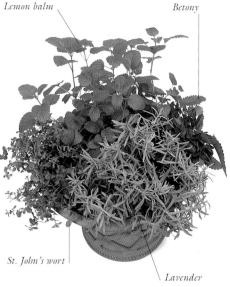

Lemon balm

Betony

St. John's wort

Lavender

4 Insert the smaller plants at the front of the container. Finish off by filling with more soil mix around the plants, leaving 1in (2.5cm) below the rim for watering. Gently firm in the plants by pressing the soil mix with the tips of your fingers.

5 Label the plants in the finished container, and water the container well with a fine-holed watering can. Make sure that the water reaches the soil mix and does not just stream off the leaves. Water twice a day for the first week after planting.

MAKING REMEDIES

Herbal remedies are easy to make using standard kitchen equipment. As well as taking advantage of the growing season's abundance to make fresh remedies, you can store up remedies for the winter months when many plants will be dormant.

GATHERING AND STORING

Gather herbs on a sunny day and when completely dry. Pick flowers when fully open and aerial parts when flowers begin to show. Harvest roots and bulbs in autumn when the pot is emptied. Dry as much as you can. Fresh herbs can also be kept in plastic bags for a short time in the freezer.

DRYING

Like vegetables, herbs are best used fresh, but they can be dried and then stored in airtight containers away from direct sunlight for later use. Most herbs will keep in this way for up to six months. When using dried herbs, remember to use half the quantity recommended for fresh herbs.

Flowers

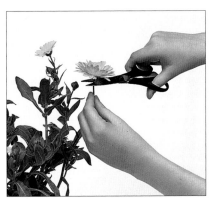

1 Pinch off, or use scissors to cut off, dry unblemished flowerheads at noon when the flowers are fully open. If picking pot marigold flowers, make sure that the green cup around each flower is retained.

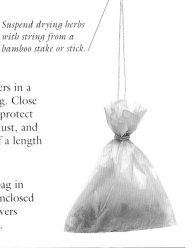

Suspend drying herbs with string from a bamboo stake or stick.

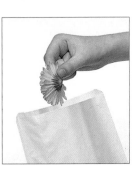

2 Place the flowers in a clean paper bag. Close the top loosely to protect the flowers from dust, and tie with the end of a length of string or twine.

3 Hang up the bag in a warm, airy, enclosed place until the flowers have become crisp.

Leaves and aerial parts

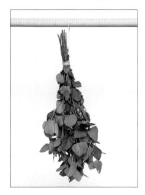

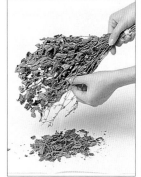

1 Pick several stalks with fresh leaves. Tie the stalks together. Hang the bunch upside down in a dry, airy place, out of direct sunlight.

2 When the leaves have dried out and are crisp, strip them off the stalks on to a flat piece of cardboard. Crumble up the leaves.

3 Place in a dark, airtight jar and store. Very moist leaves such as comfrey, borage, and plantain are best dried slowly in a warm oven for about two hours, then crumbled and stored.

Seed

In autumn, seed can be collected for use in herbal remedies and to propagate annuals such as chamomile and pot marigold. Cut off the flower stalk when the seed has formed and is desiccated. To collect the seed, hang the stalks upside down over a tray. Alternatively, a paper bag can be tied around the bunch of stalks to catch the seed.

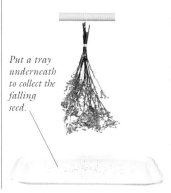

Put a tray underneath to collect the falling seed.

Roots

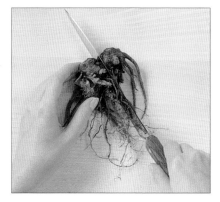

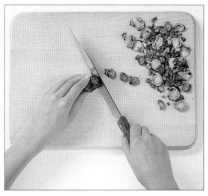

1 After removing the root from the plant, soak in cold water for about one hour to remove soil and dirt. Scrub clean. Cut through large roots and trim off excess.

2 Cut into small pieces on a chopping board. Place in a paper bag. Keep in a warm, airy place until thoroughly dried. Store in an airtight container.

TEA

Also called an infusion or tisane, a tea
is a simple way of using fresh or dried
herbs in remedies or tonics. Herbal
teas can be drunk hot or cold and can

be kept for 24 hours. For a standard
tea, use two teaspoons of fresh leaves
or flowers or one teaspoon of dried
herbs to each cup of boiling water.

1 Put fresh sprigs or leaves or some dried
plant material (see below) into a teapot
and pour over boiling water. Let steep for
at least 10 mins.

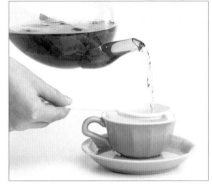

*An average
teapot holds
about 1 pint
(600ml).*

2 Place a tea strainer over
a cup to catch the steeped
herbs and pour. Strain the rest
of the tea; store in a cool place.

*To avoid contamination
from tannin, use different
teapots for herbal and
Indian tea.*

One cup infusion

A single cup of tea can be made
either in a special tisane cup (below)
or by using a tea strainer over a cup.

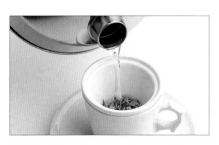

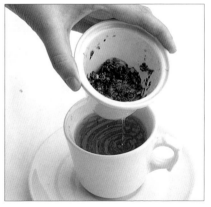

1 Place the strainer over the cup. Put a
teaspoon of dried herbs in the strainer
and pour on freshly boiled water to fill the
cup. Place a lid over the cup and strainer.

2 Leave the fresh or dried herbs to steep
in the cup for about 10 minutes, then
carefully remove the lid and the strainer.
The tea is now ready to drink.

SYRUP

Syrup is very comforting to take and therefore a good medium for soothing remedies. Do not use honey in syrup for babies under one year old.

1 Make a tea (p.88) with 5oz (150g) herbs and 1 pint (600ml) water. Steep for 20 mins. Strain into a pan, add 1 cup (375g) sugar or honey and stir slowly over heat until syrupy.

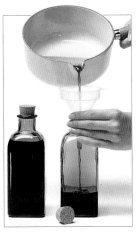

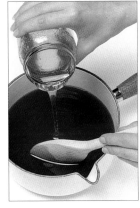

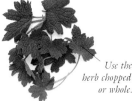

Use the herb chopped or whole.

2 Pour into glass bottles. Use cork stoppers to seal since screw-top bottles can explode if syrup ferments.

DECOCTION

Extracting the active constituents of tough plant material, such as roots and bark, requires a more vigorous action than the gentle infusion method that is used for teas and tisanes (p.88). Decoctions should be made fresh on the day of use, but they can be kept for up to 24 hours.

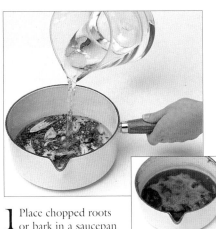

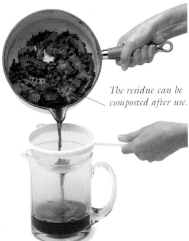

The residue can be composted after use.

1 Place chopped roots or bark in a saucepan and add cold water. Use two teaspoons of fresh, or one teaspoon of dried, herbs per cup of water. Bring to the boil; simmer for 15–20 mins. The liquid should reduce by one-third (see inset).

2 Strain the decoction through a sieve into a jug. Cover and allow the liquid to cool before drinking. Store any surplus in a cool place for use later in the day.

TINCTURE

Sometimes it is quicker and more convenient to take a spoonful of medicine than to make a tea or decoction. Tinctures are made by steeping herbs in alcohol. The alcohol extracts the active constituents of the herbs and preserves them for up to two years. Vodka is probably the best kind of alcohol to use for making tinctures because it is tasteless.

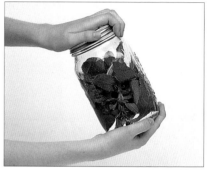

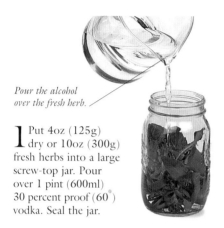

Pour the alcohol over the fresh herb.

1 Put 4oz (125g) dry or 10oz (300g) fresh herbs into a large screw-top jar. Pour over 1 pint (600ml) 30 percent proof (60°) vodka. Seal the jar.

2 Let steep in a warm place for one month. Shake the jar well every day.

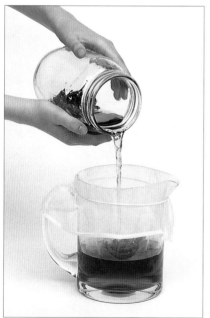

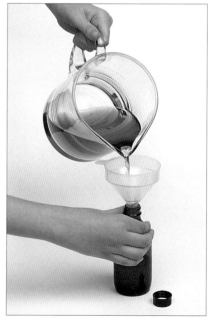

3 After a month, strain the mixture through cheesecloth into a jug. Discard or compost the remains of the herbs.

4 Pour the tincture through a funnel into a clean, dark bottle and store until the remedy is needed.

COLD INFUSED OIL

Flowers and soft parts of herbs can be made into cold infused oils. These may be used as bases for ointments (p.92) or in massage and bath oils.

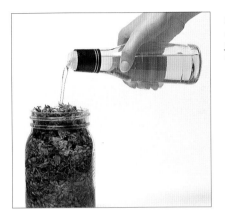

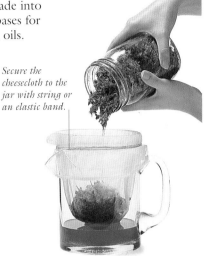

Secure the cheesecloth to the jar with string or an elastic band.

1 Fill a large screw-top jar with tightly packed flowers or leaves. Pour over enough vegetable or olive oil to cover. Screw on the lid and stand on a sunny window-sill for one month. Shake the jar daily.

2 Strain the mixture through cheese-cloth into a jug. Gather up the residue in the cloth and squeeze out remaining oil. Pour the liquid through a funnel into a dark bottle. Store in a cool, dark place.

HOT INFUSED OIL

This method of infusing oils is quicker than cold infused oils (see above) and more suitable for moist, juicy herbs such as borage. When making hot infused oil, use 1 pint (600ml) vegetable oil for 8oz (250g) of dried herbs. Infused oils can be stored in a cool, dark place for up to a year.

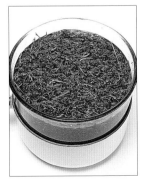

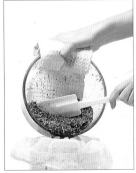

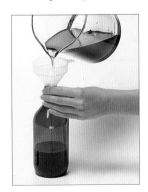

1 Place the herbs and oil in a glass bowl over a pan of simmering water.

2 Heat very gently for three hours. Strain through a muslin bag.

3 Collect the liquid in a jug and pour into a dark, sterile bottle.

OINTMENT

Ointments are made with hot or cold infused oil and beeswax, and they are good for nourishing the skin, as for diaper rash, or for strains and sprains.

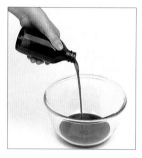
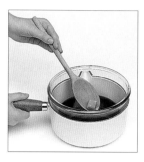
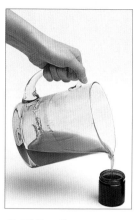

1 Pour 3½ fl oz (105ml) infused oil (p.91) into a glass bowl. Place over a saucepan of boiling water.

2 Add a ½in (1cm) square of beeswax and stir the liquid until the wax has completely melted.

3 While still warm, pour into dark ointment jars. Leave to set in a cool, dark place. Keep for up to a year.

CREAM

Creams are an emulsion of oil and water, easily absorbed by the skin. A convenient way of making it is to buy an emulsifying cream from a drugstore and heat the plant material in it.

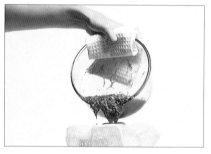

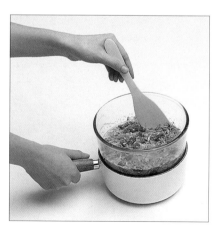

2 Remove from the heat. Strain through muslin or cheesecloth. Squeeze to extract all the liquid before the cream sets.

3 Let cool, then use a small palette knife to fill small, dark storage jars with cream. Keep for up to a year.

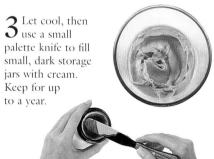

1 Melt two tablespoons of emulsifying cream over a low heat. Add two teaspoons dried or fresh herbs. Stir until cream takes on the color of the herb.

PROPAGATION CHECKLIST

The plants on pages 10–77 are listed by Latin name below. All are adaptable and most of the shrubs, subshrubs, and perennials can be left in the pot for more than one season. The easiest propagation method for each plant has been given.

Latin name	Plant type	Propagate by/from	Latin name	Plant type	Propagate by/from
Achillea millefolium	Perennial	Rooted stems	*Linum perenne*	Perennial	Seed
Agrimonia eupatoria	Perennial	Dividing	*Matricaria recutita*	Annual	Seed
Alchemilla (spp.)	Perennial	Dividing	*Medicago sativa*	Perennial	Seed
Allium sativum	Perennial	Cloves	*Melissa officinalis*	Perennial	Rooted stems
Allium schoenoprasum	Perennial	Dividing	*Mentha* x *piperita*	Perennial	Rooted stems
Allium ursinum	Perennial	Dividing	*Nepeta cataria*	Perennial	Rooted stems
Althaea officinalis	Perennial	Dividing	*Oenothera biennis*	Biennial	Seed
Arctostaphylos uva-ursi	Shrub	Cuttings	*Origanum vulgare*	Perennial	Dividing
Arnica montana	Perennial	Root cuttings	*Petroselinum crispum*	Biennial	Seed
Artemisia abrotanum	Subshrub	Cuttings	*Plantago* (spp.)	Perennial	Plantlets
Artemisia absinthium	Perennial	Dividing	*Polygonatum multiflorum*	Perennial	Root cuttings
Artemisia vulgaris	Perennial	Dividing	*Potentilla anserina*	Perennial	Plantlets
Ballota nigra	Perennial	Dividing	*Prunella vulgaris*	Perennial	Rooted stems
Baptisia australis	Perennial	Dividing	*Ranunculus ficaria*	Perennial	Dividing
Borago officinalis	Annual	Seed	*Rosa canina*	Shrub	Seed
Calendula officinalis	Annual	Seed	*Rosmarinus officinalis*	Subshrub	Cuttings
Chamaemelum nobile	Perennial	Plantlets	*Rubus idaeus*	Shrub	Suckers
Cochlearia armoracia	Perennial	Root cuttings	*Rumex crispus*	Perennial	Root cuttings
Daucus carota	Biennial	Seed	*Salvia* (spp.)	Perennial	Cuttings
Echinacea (spp.)	Perennial	Dividing	*Sanguisorba officinalis*	Perennial	Dividing
Eschscholzia californica	Annual	Seed	*Scutellaria lateriflora*	Perennial	Dividing
Eupatorium cannabinum	Perennial	Dividing	*Sempervivum tectorum*	Perennial	Plantlets
Filipendula ulmaria	Perennial	Dividing	*Silybum marianum*	Annual	Seed
Foeniculum vulgare	Perennial	Seed	*Solidago virgaurea*	Perennial	Dividing
Fumaria officinalis	Annual	Seed	*Stachys officinalis*	Perennial	Plantlets
Galega officinalis	Perennial	Seed	*Stellaria media*	Annual	Seed
Geranium robertianum	Annual	Seed	*Symphytum officinale*	Perennial	Root cuttings
Glechoma hederacea	Perennial	Rooted stems	*Tanacetum parthenium* 'Aur.'	Annual	Seed
Hamamelis virginiana	Shrub	Cuttings	*Thymus* (spp.)	Perennial	Dividing
Humulus lupulus 'Aureus'	Climber	Dividing	*Trifolium pratense*	Perennial	Plantlets
Hypericum perforatum	Perennial	Dividing	*Tropaeolum majus*	Annual	Seed
Hyssopus officinalis	Perennial	Cuttings	*Tussilago farfara*	Perennial	Root cuttings
Inula helenium	Perennial	Root cuttings	*Urtica dioica*	Perennial	Root cuttings
Iris versicolor	Perennial	Root cuttings	*Valeriana officinalis*	Perennial	Dividing
Juniperus communis	Evergreen	Cuttings	*Verbascum nigrum*	Biennial	Seed
Lamium album	Perennial	Rooted stems	*Verbena officinalis*	Perennial	Dividing
Lavandula (spp.)	Subshrub	Cuttings	*Viburnum opulus*	Shrub	Cuttings
Leonurus cardiaca	Perennial	Dividing	*Viola tricolor*	Annual	Seed

(spp.), meaning species, indicates that several species of a plant have been recommended for growing.

INDEX

Glossary

Aerial parts The parts of the plant above ground.
Anti-inflammatory Reduces inflammation.
Annual Plant that lives and dies in one year.
Antifungal Reduces growth of fungal infections.
Anti-infective Reduces growth of bacteria.
Antispasmodic Reduces spasm or cramps.
Antiseptic Inhibits growth of bacteria.
Aromatic Contains volatile oils.
Astringent Contracts organic tissue.
Biennial Takes two years to set seed, then dies.
Carminative Reduces flatulence.
Colic Spasm in the stomach or intestines.
Detoxification Process of getting rid of poisons.

Ericaceous Plant that needs acid soil.
Gelatinous Soothing, jellylike fluid.
Immune system Body's own defense system.
Inflammation Redness or swelling.
Laxative Stimulates and eases bowel action.
Mucilaginous Contains sticky, viscous sap.
Mucous membrane Tissue that secretes mucus.
Nervine Soothing nervous excitement.
Perennial Plant that produces new growth yearly.
Sedative Calms and reduces nervous tension.
Shrub Perennial plant with woody stem.
Tannin Substance that dries excess mucus.
Volatile oil Active aromatic oils in plants.

Authors' acknowledgments

The authors would like to thank Arne Herbs,
Limeburn Nurseries, Limeburn Hill, Chew
Magna, Avon BS18 8QW, and Poyntzfield
Herb Nursery, Black Isle, Dingwall, Ross-shire,
Scotland IV7 8LX.

Effie Romain would like to thank Ann Baker,
Diana Baker, Daisy Benn, Maire Cussen, Jane
Dunning, Lesley Freed, Heather Jones, Judy
Kemp, Clare Monro, Jesse Romain, and
Janet Skinner.

Sue Hawkey would like to thank Christine
Hawkey, Tom Kendall, and Simeon Smith.

Publisher's acknowledgments

Dorling Kindersley would like to thank the
following for lending pots for photography:
Amphora, Shepherd's Bush, pp.13, 33, 43 and
55; Chelsea Gardener, Chelsea, pp.25, 41 and
53; Clifton Nurseries, Little Venice, pp.17 and
63; Hode Pottery, Canterbury, pp.11, 29, 39,
49, 59 and 71; Jon Fisher, p.15; Patio Pots,
Dulwich, pp.19, 21, 31, 47 and 77. Thanks also
to Frances Richardson for hand modeling;
Karen Ward, Annette O'Sullivan, and Robert
Ford for design assistance; Sarah Ashun for
photographic assistance; Annelise Evans and
Sarah Prest for editorial assistance; Sarah Ponder
for the artworks; and Hilary Bird for the index.